From The Heart of the Lotus

FROM THE HEART OF THE LOTUS

The Teaching Stories Of Swami Kripalu

As spontaneously translated and spoken by
YOGI AMRIT DESAI

Compiled and edited by
JOHN MUNDAHL

MONKFISH BOOK PUBLISHING COMPANY
RHINEBECK, NEW YORK

Some of the photos of Swami Kripalu appearing in this book were used with the kind permission of Malay Desai. www. Amritkala.com

Library of Congress Cataloging-in-Publication Data

Kripalvanandji, Swami, 1913-1981.
  From the heart of the lotus : the teaching stories of Swami Kripalu / com-piled and edited by John Mundahl ; foreword by Rick Faulds ; preface by Amrit Desai.
    p. cm.
  ISBN 978-0-9766843-9-8
  1. Hindu stories. 2. Didactic literature. 3. Yoga. I. Mundahl, John. II. Title.
  BL1175.K68A275 2008
  294.5'432--dc22

                          2008023320

Book and cover design by Georgia Dent

Bulk purchase discounts for educational or promotional purposes are available. Contact the publisher for information.

First edition

First Impression

10 9 8 7 6 5 4 3 2 1

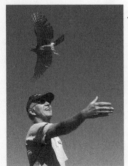

John Mundahl, compiler and editor, was a resident at the original Kripalu Yoga Ashram from 1977-1981, the four years of Swami Kripalu's stay in America. He is currently an author, retired school teacher, returned Peace Corps volunteer, yoga instructor and Ayurvedic healer. His other published work is *Tales of Courage, Tales of Dreams,* a collection of short stories. He can be reached at johnmundahl@yahoo.com or heartofthelo-tus.blogspot.com

Monkfish Book Publishing Company
27 Lamoree Road
Rhinebeck, New York 12572

Dedicated with love to Swami Kripalu, Bapuji, who told us only a lit candle can light an unlit candle.

You were my lit candle.

(John Mundahl)

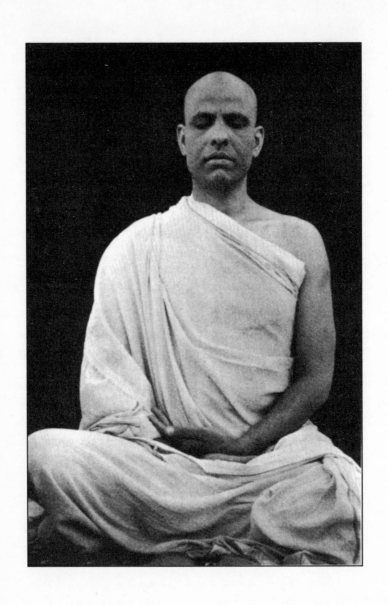

TABLE OF CONTENTS

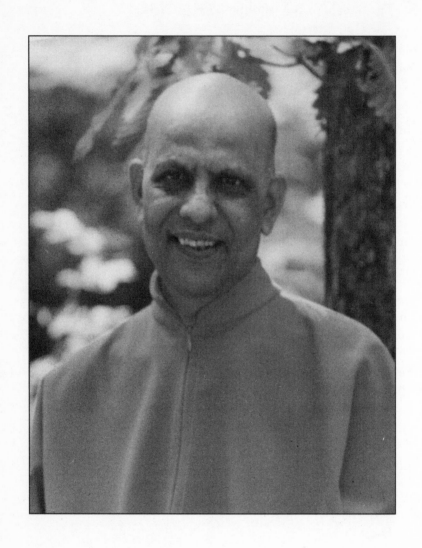

THE ANTHOLOGY OF STORIES you hold in your hand were told by a remarkable yet little known spiritual teacher who played a pivotal role in the transmission of yoga to America. Born in 1913 and raised in a rustic village, Swami Kripalu's life was a bridge connecting mystical India with the scientific and secular West.

At the tender age of nineteen, Swami Kripalu came under the tutelage of a mysterious guru who recognized his potential and personally schooled him in the yogic scriptures. Instructed to commence an intensive yoga practice later in life, Swami Kripalu spent his next decade as a music teacher and playwright. A relentless spiritual longing led the 29 year old Swami Kripalu to take monastic vows, and he began traveling on foot from village to village. The insightful spiritual discourses he gave were peppered with captivating stories, and his inspired singing stirred deep feelings within the hearts of listeners. The shopkeepers would all close their stores, creating a holiday atmosphere that enabled the entire village to be with Swami Kripalu.

During his nine years as a wandering monk, Swami Kripalu's renown grew steadily. He received many large donations from wealthy devotees, with which he established temples, libraries, and schools all over Western India. More than eloquence, talent or even good works, it was Swami Kripalu's genuine love for people that set him apart. Held dear by countless villagers, esteemed by people of influence, Swami Kripalu was widely considered a humanitarian saint.

Swami Kripalu's spiritual longing, however, was not satisfied by scriptural knowledge or the increasing status he enjoyed. At the age of 38, Swami Kripalu embarked on the practice of yoga. For the next twenty-eight years, he spent ten hours a day in focused spiritual practice, seldom leaving his meditation room despite frequent requests to travel and teach. Twelve of these years were spent in complete silence. It was during this prolonged period of seclusion that Swami Kripalu became a spiritual adept, realizing the potential glimpsed by his boyhood teacher.

It was a 66 year-old Swami Kripalu who stunned his Indian devotees by announcing his upcoming four month trip to America. After visiting disciples in California and Canada, Swami Kripalu took up residence in the Pennsylvania ashram of Yogi Amrit Desai, where Swami Kripalu resumed his life of spiritual practice, scriptural study, devotional music, and teaching. Four months turned into four years, and Swami Kripalu's presence galvanized the growth of the Kripalu Yoga community. Thousands of Americans, myself included, found him a profound and life-changing teacher.

My story of meeting Swami Kripalu is like many I've heard over the years, although to me it remains a singular and astonishing event. In the spring of 1981, after striding across the stage to receive my college diploma, I got in my car and drove directly to the Kripalu Yoga ashram, a young man on a spiritual quest. Much to my parents' dismay, the impact of four years of academic study on my developing psyche paled in comparison to my forays into the burgeoning world of American spirituality. Something in me was waking up, and I was drawn to anything that promised to expand my horizons.

More than anything else, I was fascinated by the teachings and techniques of yoga. I learned the classic yoga postures, mostly from books, and did them daily. After two years of steady practice, I sensed their transformative power and wanted to go deeper. Winding down the gravel road to the rural Kripalu retreat, I wondered what it would be like to meet a yoga master in the flesh.

No amount of practice could have prepared me for that encounter. As the 69 year-old Swami Kripalu walked into the room, my mind was catapulted into a state of focused awareness deeper than anything I'd ever experienced. My first startled thought was that he looked surprisingly like my grandfather, who was also bald and pencil thin. But the similarities ended there. Swami Kripalu was a lightning bolt wrapped in an orange robe.

The energy that emanated from Swami Kripalu was palpable, an amalgam of intimate love and sheer spiritual power. His facial expressions and gestures were mesmerizing to watch, shifting back and forth between child-like playfulness and stern truth telling. They enabled him to capture the attention and communicate with the hundred or so people gathered without saying a word. A chant started and the room became drunk on his energy. Most people got giddy with laughter and danced with joyous abandon. Some sobbed quietly. A few fell into trance and lost all outward consciousness.

A line formed and people began to approach Swami Kripalu two-by-two on their knees to receive his audience and blessing. I watched spell bound, as the impact of his silent presence on each individual was so apparent. When my turn came to make eye contact and bow before him, I discovered why. A stream of energy passed between us, and it seemed that he read my most intimate thoughts more clearly than if I had uttered them aloud. The experience was not all sweetness and light, as he saw deep into the shadowy areas of my psyche, registering the guilt, shame, and self-doubt that I covered over with a young adult bravado. While I felt exposed and vulnerable, Swami Kripalu's response was a warm and knowing acceptance that was difficult for me to take in. It reverberated in me for weeks and months, plunging me into a deep existential crisis and ultimately pulling me out the other side a significantly changed person, someone fit to embark on the spiritual path.

It was clear that Swami Kripalu was not doing anything in particular to make all this happen. He appeared relaxed and content to just be himself. The only explanation I could come up with was that his years of yoga practice had purified his body, mind, and heart in a way that allowed the full force of his being to flow through him. Whatever the cause, the result was mind boggling. Looking back. I can say that those brief hours spent in Swami Kripalu's presence shifted the trajectory of my entire life.

Swami Kripalu returned to India and died a few short months after our meeting. In the years since his death, I continued to study his teachings while deepening my involvement with the ashram community led by Yogi Desai. Swami Kripalu saw yoga as a life-long path of personal transformation. Before most of us are ready to engage with its spiritual depths, there is essential physical and psychological work to do. He called this "character building" and recommended it to anyone seeking success and fulfillment in life. For those of a mystical bent, Swami Kripalu's message remained consistent. Character building lays a foundation that makes higher realizations possible. Only a wholesome and virtuous person dedicated to something higher than his own comfort and wellbeing can scale the esoteric heights of yoga.

Swami Kripalu believed that all the world's religions reflected this same truth, emphasizing moral development as a prerequisite to initiation into their mystery schools. This is one of the reasons why stories and parables are a universal teaching tool. A story allows an inspiring message to be conveyed to a mass of people effectively, making the benefits of virtue and good character obvious by showing their results in practical life situations. On a deeper level, stories enable a masterful teacher to convey secrets of the transformative process, encoded symbolically and available to anyone willing to ponder them carefully.

All of us owe a debt to John Mundahl and Monkfish Publishing, for Swami Kripalu was a masterful teacher and these are magical stories with multiple meanings. This is spiritual literature well-worth preserving and publishing. Along with transmitting an experience of Swami Kripalu's charm and insight, they are potent seeds that can help us sprout into a fuller expression of who each of us is meant to be.

Interestingly, the stories of encounters with Swami Kripalu didn't stop with his death. Just last week, I received a letter from a person struck by a tiny photo of him in Yoga Journal magazine. He began showing up in her dreams, and then her meditations. She was writing to learn more about this enigmatic man and hopefully make sense of her experience. There was not much that I could say, beyond pointing to the fact that every religion has its saints and holy intercessors. So don't be surprised if this book is an introduction to just such a personage!

Richard Faulds
Greenville, Virginia, 2008

PREFACE

TO LIVE NEAR ONE of the greatest saints of India is an experience of profound grace. Rarely does such an evolved being exist on this plane. And here he was in the spring of 1977, Swami Kripalvanandji, lovingly known as Bapuji, living among us at the spiritual community named for him. The story of his long-awaited arrival at the Kripalu Yoga Ashram in Sumneytown, Pennsylvania, is both circuitous and auspicious.

At that time, Bapuji had maintained an intense spiritual practice, 10 hours a day for 28 years. During the first 12 years, he remained in complete silence. Bapuji's patience, perseverance, faith and fearlessness were a rare demonstration of total dedication to sadhana, an experience that greatly benefited those of us privileged to live near him during this final stage of the evolution of his consciousness. To have a Kundalini Yoga Acharya of his stature in our ashram specifically to complete the highest stage of sadhana, Nirvikalpa Samadhi, was a great fortune.

However, our fortune was destined to take an even greater turn when Bapuji began to speak publicly. When Bapuji saw the sincere hunger and love for sadhana among his grandchildren, he was inspired and moved to speak. So great was the devotion he felt from our community that he began giving regular discourses on specific days of the week. Before this, he had spoken only three times a year in India on very auspicious occasions. Garnered in silence, he communicated only when necessary by writing in chalk on a slate.

Bapuji spoke to disciples for several months before resuming his total silence and seclusion. It was love alone that motivated him to speak...and speak he did! For hours, Bapuji would charm us with his animated and detailed stories, each embedded with a precious spiritual gem.

When Bapuji began to speak to us so often and so vividly, it instantly took me back to my first encounter with him. The year was 1948; he was a wandering mendicant and I was a 16 year old boy. Bapuji was traveling from village to village giving lectures on the Bhagavad Gita. I was immediately attracted to his radiance; his essence drew me toward his compassionate heart like a giant magnet. I instantly recognized his greatness and could not get enough. I would arrive early for his discourses so I could sit as close to him as possible. I would yearn for his glance or a gesture to bring him a glass of water. My love for him was so strong that after school, when others went out to play, I would race to the Goshala, where Bapuji stayed during his visits to my small town of Halol. It was a simple two-story concrete building with a covered front porch. I would wait every day for Bapuji to come so I might have the opportunity to serve him in any way. The newly awakened Kundalini was guiding him through vigorous practices of asanas and pranayamas. He would come out of his room exhausted but radiant with Shakti. By then, I became so close to him that I had the rare privilege to massage and bathe him after his emergence from his intense Kundalini Yoga meditations.

One day as Bapuji came out of his meditation room and was descending the stairs, he saw me teaching my young friends yoga postures on the lower floor. He said, "Come tomorrow and I will take you into my meditation room." I knew that an invitation to be present during his direct meditative expressions of Kundalini kriyas was rarely allowed.

The next day, I sat quietly as Bapuji began his meditation and after a time, he began what looked like yoga postures and dance-like movements performed in a deeply meditative trance-like state. When it was over, Bapuji told me that these kriyas were directly conducted by Kundalini. My young mind could not comprehend the significance of the profound impact it would have on me. It wasn't until years later, during my own spontaneous awakening, that the depth of what I had witnessed became clear. When I experienced prana kriyas myself, suddenly the memory of what I had seen in Bapuji's meditation room nearly 30 years before revealed itself to me. My own experience clarified what Bapuji had demonstrated—the divine Presence of Kundalini manifesting in a physical form.

Over the years, I became one of Bapuji's closest disciples and refrained from marrying for an additional five years at Bapuji's request, so I could focus on my yogic study and sadhana with him. Even after I came to the U.S. in 1960, I maintained my connection with Bapuji and visited him as often as I could. Each time, I would invite him to come back to the States with me for a visit, especially after the two Pennsylvania ashrams I had named in his honor began to flourish. I was always deeply inspired by Bapuji and wanted my disciples to learn directly from my guru. Each time I would ask, Bapuji would decline my request, saying, "I cannot travel until I have entered Nirvikalpa Samadhi." I had nearly given up my requests when one day while I was visiting him at Kayavarohan (the temple he built in his guru Dadaji's memory), Bapuji called for me. What he next said took me completely by surprise: "Now I will come to America with you for a few months. But I have one condition. When I am ready to return to India, you must not urge me to stay."

I truly understood Bapuji's request. He was not certain whether conditions in a foreign country would be appropriate for the delicate state of his sadhana. His practice had to be conducted in an atmosphere that was most conducive and supportive, without distractions. He also knew that if I pleaded with him to stay, his compassionate heart was so open, he would probably say 'yes' not to disappoint me.

After Bapuji declared that he would come to America, I rushed back to make adequate preparations to welcome him at our ashram. As is the protocol in the service to one's guru, I then returned to India to accompany him to America. When the Pan Am jet bearing our beloved Bapuji landed that May, we were met at JFK by a group of disciples who had fastidiously prepared for his arrival. It was a scene of great fanfare...the love between our teacher and his grandchildren, as he called them, was palpable. Bapuji took up residence in a magical cabin on the highest point of our property in the Perkiomen Valley of Pennsylvania. Situated deep in the woods and only accessible by footpath, it was a perfect abode for his sadhana.

After his arrival, he found that the ashram environment, seclusion and services were indeed most supportive. During his time with us, I was with Bapuji every day. He would share with me the different experiences he was going through in his sadhana. One day, he wrote on his slate, "Amrit, today the name you have given to my home here, Muktidham, the abode of liberation, has been truly fulfilled." I understood at that moment that he had reached the final state of complete liberation – Mukti.

In his final farewell address on September 27, 1981, he wrote, "I came to America solely for the purpose of meeting you. I imagined I would stay for only a few months, but today four and a quarter years have passed...I have stayed...it feels like 4 ¼ days. I have had the good fortune to bathe in the lake of your love and drink its waters daily. I have always experienced happiness with your selfless service. With the grace of God, I have not found any flaws in that service. I consider the collective love of every one of you as the love of the Lord Himself.

Today the long sweet dream of 4 ¼ years has come to an end. I am going into more restricted seclusion. I beg your permission to say farewell. I belong to the Lord and I sincerely pray I will always belong to Him."

To this day, the hillside cabin known as Muktidham resonates with his energy.

Just as he did back in 1948, Bapuji's animated speaking style was mesmerizing. When he spoke in story-form, it was much more than an entertaining anecdote. Like so many great masters, he taught in parables, seemingly simple stories about people, animals or insects that are actually revelations that illuminate the depth of spiritual teachings.

As he related each enchanting tale, his abrupt changes in mood, tone and facial expression were something to behold. He was both actor and author. The group would erupt in peals of laughter and dissolve into pools of tears just by the way he articulated. The fact that he was speaking in Gujarati to Americans was of no consequence. So connected were his feelings toward his English-speaking audience, his communication was more like communion on an energetic level. His speaking was beyond mere words, it was the universal language of love.

In this book, you will find a collection of stories related by Bapuji during his time in the U.S. at the Kripalu Ashram. If you read deeply into his words, imagine his animated expression and feel the depth of his wisdom, you will receive the same gift of insight and love that Bapuji gave to us directly during those precious few years.

Yogi Amrit Desai, 2008

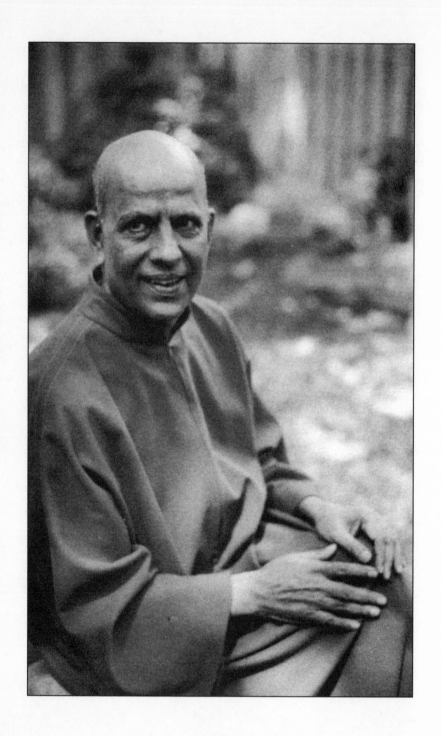

INTRODUCTION

"THE SPIRITUAL HISTORY OF India is so great that it's almost beyond description," Swami Kripalu told us once. "Even now, in India's sad state, there are still samskaras, or impressions, from this past glory. One of these customs is that a person may adopt the clothes of a swami and be taken care of by society. Today in India there are hundreds of thousands of sadhus and they are all fed, clothed, and housed by Indian society, even by the poorest of the poor.

Naturally, some abuse this system. But India believes that saints are the gems of the country, and just as it takes tons of coal to produce one diamond, it takes tons of sadhus to produce one true saint. India believes this is worthwhile. One sun in the sky is enough. It is enough for the entire world."

Swami Kripalu, or Bapuji, as we called him, could have been talking about himself when he spoke those words, although he would have burst into laughter at the thought. Born in 1913 to devote Hindu parents in the western state of Gujarat, his life was destined to end early at the age of 19, in total despair, crushed under the wheels of a train in suicide had not fate intervened. That night, while he was sobbing and saying his final prayers in a small temple in Bombay close to the railroad tracks, a Mahatma, a great soul, wearing only a loincloth, came silently into the temple and touched the sobbing youth on the shoulder and said, "Son."*

He uttered the word with such sweetness and love that Bapuji accepted him that evening as his guru and dedicated his life to him, and so began the spiritual training and spiritual ascent of one of India's greatest saints and greatest spiritual treasures. His full story is told in two beautiful books, *Pilgrim of Love* by Atma Jo-Ann Levitt, and *Infinite Grace, The Story of My Spiritual Lineage*, by Swami Rajarsi Muni.

---

* See story #30, How I Meet My Gurudev.

In 1977, at the age of 64, Bapuji stunned his huge spiritual family in India by saying he was leaving for America, for three months, promising to be back. When we heard the news at the Kripalu Yoga Ashram in Sumneytown, Pennsylvania where he would be staying, we began the frenetic preparations for his visit. Finally, on May 20th, 1977, we drove to Kennedy Airport in New York to welcome him to the United States.

Bapuji came into our waiting room first and there was a flurry of activity to make sure he was comfortable on the soft chair we had prepared for him. Then he reached for his slate and wrote us a message:

"My Dear Grandchildren. I am extremely pleased to meet you all. At present I am in such a critical stage of yoga sadhana that I cannot travel even two miles. Yet, I have come to you, traveling thousands of miles by plane. That is the miracle of your pure love."

He smiled sweetly, unfazed by the long exhausting flight from India, his face loose and alive, the picture of a doting grandfather. But then he looked my way and suddenly a movie ignited inside my forehead, in color, and I became aware of his immense spiritual power. The pictures came quickly. It was a scene from my childhood. I was 14 years old. I had just broken my left arm in gym class. During the operation, much to my surprise, I had floated above my body near the ceiling over the operating table and watched the doctor straighten out my arm. He straightened it by pulling it in two different directions at once, and then casually talked about his golf game. "Well, it looks like I'll miss my tee time!" He laughed.

I was confused and terrified. I didn't know if I was alive or dead. Then a bald headed man in an orange robe came to me. "Don't be afraid," he said, in thought, not words, and all fear vanished. As he floated away, I tried to follow. "No,"he said with compassion, "You can't come. But I'll see you again when you start yoga." I had never heard of the word yoga before and soon forgot the incident.

And now here he was again, the same bald headed man in an orange robe! I tried to check my tears. "You can't cry like this in front of everyone!" But then I looked around and everyone else was crying, too, so I just kept crying.

Two days later, in a dream, there was an explosion at the base of my spine. It blew me 50 feet into the air where I floated giddy with bliss. Then a voice said, "Look down." I looked down and saw my body going through one yoga posture after another with effortless grace. Then the voice said. "When the prana in the body of the seeker is awakened, all postures happen automatically."

That's how I met Bapuji. My meeting, though unique to me, was no more dramatic than anyone else's who met him. Invariably he hid his spiritual power. He was totally content to be just our grandfather. On his first Father's Day with us, he said, "I love you so much that I just want to pick you all up and place you on my lap!"

Bapuji stayed with us for four years. He loved it here. He found peace and solitude at Muktidam, the house in the woods above our ashram in Sumneytown where he did the final four years of his beloved yoga sadhana.*

During the first three months of his stay, he broke his silence and spoke to us twice a day. Except for formal birthday discourses, he spoke spontaneously on a wide range of spiritual topics. His talks were full of stories! He couldn't speak on any subject without telling a story! He was a playwright in India and loved drama and often would change his voice to fit the characters in the story, and then he would laugh and cry along with us as he told the story. Once he laughed so hard he fell over! And it was at one of his own stories!

This book is a collection of the stories he told us. I've collected all I could find, 102. If you live at the Kripalu Center, or if you visit the Kripalu Center, or if you're a Kripalu Yoga teacher, or if you're simply curious about his life, know that Swami Kripalu was a great man. He was full of joy and compassion. He had and still has, immense spiritual power, and if you open your heart to him while you read these stories, perhaps he will come to you.

As insignificant as I often feel in the grand scheme of things, Bapuji still comes to me. The last time he appeared was a year ago

---

* Muktidam is now a shrine and is open to visitors.

when I was collecting these stories. One evening I was saying japa, mantra repetition using beads. My mind was distracted and I quit early. That night Bapuji came to me in a dream. He floated in from the left, his arms motionless as he moved. I could only see his upper body. He was youthful and radiant. He placed my mala beads in my hand and then he placed his hand over mine and showed me how to do japa again, patiently one bead at a time with great love. Then he smiled and wagged his head from side to side and floated away.

I awoke with a start and burst into tears.

"Remember me! Remember me! Don't forget me!" I burbled and sobbed out loud, not caring anymore if anyone heard me. But all was silent in the room, just the darkness of the night, and I knew better than to try and follow him, although that was all I wanted to do and all I will ever want to do.

John Mundahl
Mounds View, Minnesota
2008

My Beloved Child
Break your heart no longer
Each time you judge yourself
You break your own heart.
You stop feeding on the love,
Which is the wellspring of your vitality
The time has come. Your time
To live
To celebrate
And to see the goodness that you are.
You my child are divine
You are pure
You are sublimely free
You are god in disguise
And you are always perfectly safe.
Do not fight the dark,
Just turn on the light.
Let go
And Breathe into the goodness that you are.

Swami Kripaluanandadji
(Bapuji)

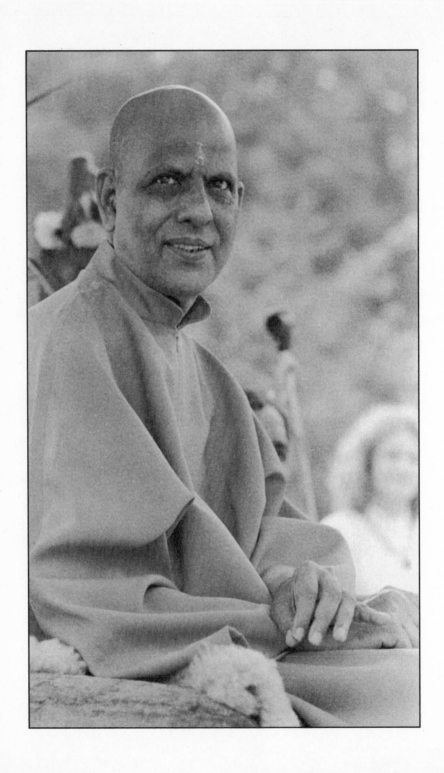

The first requisite in life is that peace reign in our household. To establish peace in our household we will have to win the hearts of every individual, big or small. When peace is established by force it isn't peace, but a regime of terror. Divinity is born out of the peace founded on love. Peace and tolerance are born when we learn to control our mind and emotions. We should try to deal with every family member with love. If we seldom consider the feelings of others and only concern ourselves with our own state of mind, disagreements, friction, and dissatisfaction are born. If we are agreeable with others, they become agreeable with us. Instill the love of God into your family. Without surrender and service, love cannot evolve.

THE DISTRACTED HUSBAND

ONCE THERE WAS A scientist who spent all day totally involved in his research work. He couldn't remember if he ate lunch, or took a shower. After observing this strange behavior, his wife decided to intervene. When it was time for his shower, she went into his study, took him by the hand, and without uttering a single word, gestured to him to get up. The unexpected visit startled him, and with great surprise he recognized that it was his wife. He laughed and asked her sweetly.

"What do you want me to do?"

She didn't say a thing. But like one leading a blind man, she led him to the shower.

"I've already showered!" He said.

"You showered yesterday, not today," his wife replied.

At lunchtime, when she took him to the dining room, he again expressed his surprise.

"Why have you served me this meal twice?" He asked.

"Yesterday you fasted; you didn't eat anything," she replied. "It's noon now, and this is the first meal you've been served."

"Thank you. Thank you. You're taking good care of me," he said. He affectionately tapped her on the shoulder and expressed his pleasure.

A few days later, his wife took him to the dining room and left him after serving his lunch. Some friends came to visit her and they spent two hours talking. When she returned to the dining room, her husband was writing something on a piece of paper. He had forgotten to eat his lunch.

Upon seeing this, she became angry and snatched the pen and paper away from him. "How strange you are!" She said, scolding him. "Your lunch is cold and now I have to reheat it."

He looked at his wife's angry face and at his meal. He understood the situation and he acknowledged his offense. Then he took his plate of food and put it on his wife's head.

"What are you doing?" She asked. She thought it was some sort of joke.

"I'm warming my lunch," her husband replied. "Your anger is so hot that my lunch will be warm in a short time."

She burst into laughter and her anger melted away.

To love is to suffer. When love becomes tolerant, fragrance spreads from it and the heart of the beloved overflows with joy. If the lover can't tolerate the anger of the beloved, then that love is about to be shattered.

STORY #2

Compassion is the religion of the Lord, the religion of love, and the religion of everyone. The brother of compassion is service, not obligation, and service is selfless. The daughter of non-violence is compassion. The daughter of violence is cruelty. The pain of others doesn't touch everyone. Those touched by the pain of others are God's messengers because God can comfort his suffering children through them.

THE OLD MASTER WHIPS THE YOUNG PRINCE

ONCE THERE WAS AN old acharya, an old spiritual teacher. He was an exceptional saint and an exceptional teacher. He served the king of that area and the king respected him so much that he never disobeyed an order from this saint, even though he himself was the king.

The king had one son.

One day the king called the old master to his side and said, "I'm getting old. The prince is ready to sit upon the throne. I'd like to have a coronation ceremony. Please plan this in keeping with the scriptures."

The acharya planned the ceremony with the help of others in the court, and when the festive day arrived, everyone in the kingdom celebrated. That morning the king and queen inspected the special clothes that the prince was to wear, along with the jewelry and ornaments.

"Everything is fine," the king said. "Bathe and dress the prince now for the ceremony."

But when the prince was only half dressed, he received a message from the acharya. The message said come at once to see me.

The prince was surprised. What could be so important that his teacher would call him now? The prince left immediately because he, too, never disobeyed an order from this great saint. Maybe

Guruji wants to tell me something special, the young prince thought, since this is such an important day in my life.

The prince entered the acharya's room and bowed to him. Immediately the acharya took a whip off the wall and whipped him hard on his bare back! Then he did it four more times! He whipped him so hard there were marks and blood on his back.

The prince screamed with pain!

"Why is Guruji punishing me?" He asked himself. "Normally Guruji is gentle and explains everything to me! Today he's punishing me severely and yet saying nothing! I must have made some mistake!"

When the beating was over, the young prince stood up and looked into the face of his teacher. The old acharya's face was peaceful, totally balanced and calm, and full of compassion for the young prince.

The attendants rushed out to tell the king and soon the king and queen and many others arrived. Here it was, such a happy day, full of music and dancing, and yet the prince was being beaten? No one could understand this.

The prince left the room and everyone saw the marks and blood on his back. They saw the pain and hurt on his face and the tears in his eyes. They knew he had an innocent nature, yet no one dared say a word, not even the king. The old acharya was loved and respected so much that no one ever doubted the wisdom of his actions.

Everyone returned inside the palace and the great coronation ceremony continued. By the end of the day, the young prince had become the new king.

"Maharaja," the old acharya said to the young prince the next day. "Now you're the king, so I'll call you Maharaja. Now you must serve as final Judge on all matters in the kingdom. So I ask you to administer justice to me for the harsh beating I gave you yesterday."

The young king became silent.

"Why did you punish me?" He asked softly

"I saw the need for it," the old acharya said.

"Did I commit some wrong?" the young king asked. "Did I make a mistake?"

"No, you did nothing wrong," the old acharya said.

"Then why did you punish me?" The young king asked.

"To teach you a lesson," the old acharya said.

"What is the lesson?" The young king asked.

"You were born into the family of a king. You were raised with great love. You have never experienced physical punishment. Now you're the king and you must pass judgment on others. I wanted you to know the pain of physical punishment so that you don't rule too harshly. You must punish people with understanding."

The young king stood up and bowed to his teacher.

"Guruji," he said softly. "I know the horrible pain of the whip now and I won't be unjust to anyone."

"May you rule with compassion," the old acharya said, and then he left the room.

STORY #3

The dharma of service is the dharma of love, the very embodiment of love. In whomever love arises, divine vision also arises, so that service does not remain inaccessible to him. The person who becomes the embodiment of love does not remain an ordinary human being. His faults are transformed into strengths and he becomes an extraordinary person.

THE SAINT AND THE SCORPION

IT WAS 8:00 O'CLOCK in the morning. Countless pilgrims were bathing in the holy waters of the Ganges. Among them was an aged ascetic saint who had dunked himself five times, reciting each time, "Ganga Hara. Praise to Lord Shiva and the Holy River Ganges."

Before the saint had finished bathing, however, he saw a scorpion drowning in the river. His tender heart was filled with compassion.

"That poor scorpion," he thought. "It's going to die."

He knew the scorpion was poisonous and would definitely sting him if he touched it. But being a true lover of religion, he fearlessly approached the scorpion, lifted it into his cupped hands, and swiftly and skillfully threw it toward the riverbank.

The scorpion immediately stung him.

The saint's hand burst into flames, but he ignored the excruciating pain. The scorpion fell short of the riverbank, though, because the sting had taken strength from the saint's hand.

Quickly the saint approached the scorpion again. This time there were pilgrims watching from the riverbank.

"Reverend saint!" they called. "What are you doing? Let it die! What's the purpose of saving it?"

The saint said nothing.

He took the scorpion into his cupped hands a second time and threw it toward the river bank. The scorpion stung him again.

The painful flames already blazing in his hands were made worse by the second sting. Yet the saint ignored the discomfort again; he was an ascetic, an embodiment of tolerance itself. Sighs slipped from the mouths of the people on the bank.

"Reverend saint!" they cried again. "Why are you making this useless effort? Even though the scorpion is almost dead, it hasn't given up its instinct to sting!"

Once again, the saint said nothing.

The scorpion was still not on shore, so the saint waded a third time over to the scorpion, scooped it up into his cupped hands and threw it toward the shore.

The scorpion delivered a third ungrateful sting. But at last, the saint's efforts were successful. His eyes flooded with joy and his lips formed a sweet smile. Then he turned to the pilgrims on the riverbank and said,

"If this poisonous creature hasn't renounced its instinct to sting, even at the threat of impending death, why should I, a saint, renounce my instinct to serve living beings?"

STORY #4

Non-stealing is the fifth discipline prescribed by Patanjali and is defined in the scriptures as not desiring anyone's wealth by thought, word, or deed, and not taking anyone's possessions, no matter how small, without their permission. When we obtain what we desire by honest means, our mind remains at peace, free of fear. When we obtain what we desire by dishonest means, we lose our peace of mind and become victims of fear.

DALA TARVADI AND THE EGGPLANTS

THERE ONCE WAS A man named, Dala Tarvadi. He lived in a small village. He had read a few religious scriptures. One day, with no particular purpose in mind, Tarvadi took a walk to the outskirts of the village. He noticed a small garden owned by a man named, Vashrambhai. Tarvadi decided to walk over to see what Vashrambhai had planted. In the distance, he saw Vashrambhai tending his garden.

"Vashrambhai!" Tarvadi called out loudly, "How are you today?"

"I'm fine," Vashrambhai replied casually. "What brings you out this way, Tarvadi?"

"I had a little work at the outskirts of the village," Dala Tarvadi said. "I happened to see your garden and thought I would go see what you've planted. What did you plant this year?"

"Vegetables," replied Vashrambhai. He took Dala Tarvadi on a tour of the entire garden. Then he said, "Here, take home a few of these eggplants; they're wonderful."

Tarvadi gratefully took the eggplants and went home. That evening he prepared the eggplants for supper and liked them very much. Two or three days later, he remembered those delicious eggplants again, but he knew that Vashrambhai wouldn't give them away free again. Yet, he didn't want to pay the expensive price for them, either.

Engrossed in thoughts about the eggplants, once again Dala Tarvadi walked to the outskirts of the village. He looked around to make sure that the orchard was empty. Then he trespassed into the garden and went to the small mound where the eggplants were growing. But just as he was about to take some eggplants, he remembered a line from the scriptures:

"If you take anything without the owner's permission, you're stealing."

Tarvadi knew that the owner wasn't around and that even if he was, he wouldn't just give away expensive eggplants for nothing. He wrestled with his conscience for a few minutes, and eventually devised a way to take the eggplants without cost, and still feel that he was observing the scriptures.

"Oh, Garden! Sister, Garden!" He called.

But how could a garden of vines, vegetables, and trees give a response? It couldn't, of course, so Dala Tarvadi spoke in reply for the garden in a sweet, feminine voice.

"What do you want, Dala Tarvadi?" He had the garden say.

"May I take two or three eggplants?" Tarvadi asked in his own voice.

"Sure, my brother," he had the garden say, in the same feminine voice. "Help yourself. Take ten or eleven." Immediately Dala Tarvadi helped himself to eleven eggplants.

After learning the exact time at which Vashrambhai went home and the garden would be empty for the day, Tarvadi began to come for eggplants every evening.

Eventually, Vashrambhai realized that someone was stealing his eggplants. So one day he hid in the garden when he normally would have gone home. Soon, he spied Dala Tarvadi come and pick eggplants in his usual manner, talking to the garden first, and then taking eggplants when he had permission from the garden. Vashrambhai came out from his hiding place and caught him.

Dala Tarvadi was embarrassed and ashamed, but Vashrambhai didn't scold or hit him. Instead, he tied a rope around Tarvadi and lowered him into the well. When the water came up to Tarvadi's neck, Vashrambhai called out,

"Brother Well! Oh, Brother Well!"

Then Vashrambhai changed his voice and spoke for the well.

"Yes, Vashrambhai, my brother! Did you call me? What do you want?"

"Shall I dunk this man two or three times?"

"Dunk him ten or eleven times, my good brother!"

So, with the consent of the well, Vashrambhai dunked Dala Tarvadi eleven times before pulling him out of the well. When Dala Tarvadi was exhausted and almost unconscious from swallowing water, Vashrambahi pulled him out. Tarvadi pulled himself together and went home with wet clothes, ashamed of his actions. He had learned his lesson and from that day on, he gave up his habit of stealing eggplants!

Anyone can write or speak religious thoughts, but not everyone can practice them. Religious behavior requires discipline and anyone who can't consistently practice discipline can't absorb religion.

STORY #5

Usually what we call love isn't love. True love never ends. Once the flame of true love is lit, it can never be put out. It doesn't start and stop, sometimes on, sometimes off. It's always giving and serving, no matter what. This is it's nature. One who can't tolerate pain can't travel on the path of true love. True love is for fools. They are fools to the desires of the world, so worldly people call them fools. But they aren't fools, really. They're simply full of love. Close your eyes and draw all your senses inward and enter the depth of your heart and ask yourself: Have I ever experienced this kind of love from anybody? It's so rare.

THE LORD'S ONE WISH

ONCE TWO SAINTS WERE standing in heaven. They were new to heaven. They had just arrived. One saint was young and the other was old. There was a large highway next to where they were standing.

"Son," the old saint said, "Watch this highway for awhile with me."

Soon a large procession passed by in front of them. There was one great master in front followed by thousands of people.

"Who's that supreme leader?" The young saint asked.

"His name is Sadguru Shantiji," the old saint said. "He was a true teacher on earth. Look how many people he has brought home to the Lord."

The procession passed. Then another procession began. It was a bit smaller, but it was still quite large. Another great master was leading this procession.

"Who's the leader of this procession?" The young saint asked.

"His name is Sadguru Anandaji," the old saint said. "He, too, was a true teacher on earth. Look how many people he has brought home to the Lord."

This continued for seven processions. Each procession was led by a great master.

Finally, the last procession came by. There were only two people in the procession.

"Why are there only two people in this procession?" The young saint asked with great surprise. "And who is that poor saint with only one follower?"

"That's the Lord," the old saint said. "He loves us so much that His one wish is that we all grow up and become greater than Him. See how He keeps His new son close? Someday that son, too, will have a large following."

Can a father really be smaller than his son? Yes, when there's true love the father is always smaller than his son. The father is the seed and the son is the tree, which is always bigger. The father's one wish is: "Son, grow. Grow from a seed into a tree."

STORY #6

We all must battle anger. Anger is a powerful distraction to the mind and we must overcome it if we're to arrive at lasting peace. Anger may visit us from our external surroundings or at any moment from within our own minds. When these thoughts arise, there's no switch to shut them off, but one trick is to start a new train of thought that doesn't disturb us so much. Devotees in India use pictures and statues for this. Westerns may think that this is idol worship, but it isn't. The pictures and statues create such a loving response from the devotee, that the devotee's mind is washed in love and becomes one-pointed and ready to pray and meditate.

THE ANGRY YOUNG SWAMI

ONCE THERE WAS A young swami. He was offering prayers one evening in a small temple. He was dressed in saffron clothes and had a shaved head and carried only a small prayer cloth and a water pot. Dutifully he placed his prayer cloth on the floor of the temple and began his evening prayers.

Soon a woman entered. She entered quickly and without intention walked across his prayer cloth.

"How awful!" The young swami said to himself. He got very angry. "How disrespectful of this woman! She walked across my cloth while I was sitting for evening prayers and then walked away without a word of apology!"

The young swami continued his prayers and then got up to leave. By chance the woman finished her prayers at the same time and was also leaving.

"Come here!" The young swami called. He was still angry. "You walked across my prayer cloth and disturbed my evening prayers!"

The woman was totally surprised.

"And what were you doing looking at a woman while you were praying?" She asked. "Aren't you a swami? Were you really praying? How could you see me if you were really praying? Now I'll tell you what I was doing and why this happened. This is my favorite temple. I come here everyday. When I see the statue of the Lord in this temple, my mind fills with love and I forget about everything, even where I am. I never saw you. I only saw the Lord."

The young swami knelt and touched the feet of the woman and all anger left him.

STORY #7

The Goddess of Compassion has a vast kingdom in India. This doesn't mean that she doesn't reign in other countries, but a special characteristic of India is that beggars can extend their hand to anyone. Their begging is not prohibited. In this way, compassion has the special characteristic that enables one to practice compassion even when one deserves compassion. We are suffering and others are suffering, too. Those in pain should help others in pain.

THE BEGGAR WOMAN'S COMPASSION

ONCE UPON A TIME in India, there was a young beggar woman named, Malti, who used to wander through a large city. Every night she slept beneath a tree, or on the side of the road. Malti never married, although once she lived with a beggar for a few months and had a son by him.

Unlike other beggars, she didn't ask people for food. She was in such need, however, that just seeing her was enough to melt anyone's heart. Occasionally, a sister gave her an old sari. Another sister gave her a meal. Other sisters would ask,

"Malti, are you hungry? Have you eaten today?"

"Ma'am," Malti would reply lovingly, "Today I have eaten four giant sweetballs given to me by Savitabahen. When I asked for rice and soup, she told me: Eat these nice sweetballs today. You can have the rice and dahl tomorrow."

When it got late in the day and Malti hadn't eaten, she would stand in the street a little longer. If no one offered her food, she would stand in the courtyard of a generous sister. When the sister came out, Malti would address her by name, as she knew the names of many sisters. She would always add, "Ma'am," after calling their names

"Have you eaten today?" The women would ask

"I would accept some food if you have any extra," Malti would reply hesitantly.

Immediately she would be given food. Quite often, she helped a sister with her chores, as if she were a member of the woman's family.

One day, Malti found a 24-carat gold necklace. She took the necklace to a lady and gave it to her saying,

"Ma'am, I found this necklace while walking down the street. Please try to find the owner."

After this incident, the people in the city loved her even more.

Malti's shelter was the canopy of a huge banyan tree. She tied ropes to the branches and made a hammock where she rocked her son. When she hummed a song and rocked her son, the expression on her face was total contentment. Her face glistened with the same happiness of a rich woman.

During the winter, she slept in the courtyard of a ruined inn.

This is how she lived. Her entire year would pass in this way. In spite of wearing old, torn clothes, in spite of having no home, property, or household articles, Malti didn't feel like she lacked anything. She was happy.

One morning, Malti woke up a bit earlier than usual. It was still dark, as the sun hadn't fully risen. She knew her way well enough along the path, however, to perform her morning duties. While washing her hands and feet in a small nearby creek, she heard the sound of a child crying. She was greatly surprised for she knew there were no homes in the area.

"Has some other beggar woman like me come here this morning with her child?" She said to herself.

She looked around, but saw no one. Then she walked in the direction of the crying child and came to a small bridge over the creek. Tucked under the bridge, near the water, she spied a small bag. Inside was a crying newborn infant. She looked around again, but there was no one else in sight.

"This must be the child of a widow," she said to herself, "Or maybe the child of an unwed mother, someone who has abandoned it."

She gently touched the helpless baby girl. When their eyes met, the baby stopped crying. Malti took the infant in her lap and caressed her affectionately from head to toe. She kissed the child on both cheeks, and began to nurse her. Many times Malti hadn't eaten a single crumb of food for three days, yet she had never shed a tear over her condition. But now, at the sight of this helpless infant girl, a cloudburst of tears gushed from her eyes.

She returned to her shelter with the baby, and within a few days, Malti had already forgotten that this was an abandoned child that no one had wanted. She accepted the child as the blessed gift of the Lord, and she loved her baby girl and boy equally.

A few days later, Malti was standing on a familiar street hoping to receive food.

"Malti," some of the women asked, "Where did you get that baby girl?"

"The Lord gave her to me," Malti replied briefly, lowering her head.

"We don't understand," The sisters remarked, "God gave her to you?"

"Yes," Malti said, and then she explained that someone had abandoned the infant, and that she had found the baby crying desperately under a bridge.

"I found the infant, and fearing that dogs or other wild animals would kill her, I brought her home."

Everyone was deeply touched by Malti's compassion.

"This isn't a beggar woman," they said. "This is the Goddess of Compassion."

Those with great wealth are considered rich. Yet if despite their wealth they aren't generous, they're really paupers, because they behave like paupers. Conversely, those who are poor but who are generous despite their poverty, are actually wealthy, because they behave like wealthy people. We can all give generously whether we're rich or poor. To equate charity solely with gifts of money, clothes, or food is delusion. We can give countless other gifts such as education, security, and comfort. The Lord is invoked in our hearts whenever our hearts melt at the sight of a helpless person's intolerable pain.

STORY #8

Many people come to the saints seeking peace. "How can I find peace?" They ask. This question has been with us forever and ever. Our restless minds are the cause of the disturbance, and to bring our minds back to rest, we must firmly let go of disturbing thoughts. Just as a baby pulls his own hair and then cries, unaware that he is causing his own pain, so too we hold on to our destructive thoughts and then cry in pain. To become peaceful, we must stay awake and firmly practice thought control.

THE DEMANDING DAUGHTER

ONCE THERE WAS A rich businessman who had only one daughter. When she grew to be a young woman, her parents thought she should be married. Their daughter, however, was spoiled. Being an only child, she had been raised with a great deal of attention, and now she was used to it. In fact, she demanded it.

"We think it's time for you to get married," her parents told her one day. "We're searching for an appropriate husband."

"I'll definitely get married," their daughter said. "But I have one condition. Whoever I marry must allow me to hit him seven times on the head every day with my shoe. Every day, seven blows!"

"My dear daughter!" The father said, "You can't treat your husband that way!"

"Yes, I can!" The daughter argued. "Any man who can't put up with seven blows from me each day is a coward. If he's brave, can't he stand seven blows with a shoe?"

The father tried to reason with her, but she insisted.

"I'll only marry a man who will take seven blows from me with a shoe every day!" she said. "And that's final!"

The news spread to the entire town. The rich man's daughter was going to get married, but her husband would have to take seven blows from her shoe every day.

There were many poor young men in that town. They wanted to marry the daughter to get at the family money. But then they thought about the seven blows every day, and were scared off. The poorest young men in the town, however, were bolder.

"Seven blows?" they said. "That's not so bad. Even if I get seven blows every day, I'll still live better than I am now for the rest of the day." Often they approached the house of the rich man, determined to ask for the daughter's hand in marriage, but when they got close, they thought about the seven blows and ran away.

Many days and months passed. Nothing could change the girl's mind.

"I would rather stay unmarried for the rest of my life than change my mind," she said. "If I do get married, my husband has to take seven blows every day from me."

Then one day a young man came to town. He was a guest that evening in the rich man's house. He was very intelligent. The businessman liked him and thought he would be a good husband for his daughter.

Taking the young man aside, the businessman said,

"I intend to have my daughter marry soon, but I have one huge problem. My daughter agrees to marry, but only if she can hit her husband seven times every day on the head with her shoe. My daughter has no other faults, just this one. She was raised with a lot of attention, and now she demands it. Except for this, she is really much better than the other girls."

The young man met the girl and saw that she was smart and beautiful. But he wondered why she insisted on hitting her husband over the head?

After thinking about this for a long time, he spoke with the father.

"I would like to marry your daughter," he said. "And it's not for money."

The father was delighted and the marriage day was fixed.

On the day of the wedding, the entire town turned out. Everyone carefully looked at the young man who dared to marry this girl, and felt sorry for him. This man was really going to suffer!

Before the marriage ceremony began, the girl reminded her father,

"Do you remember my one condition?"

"Yes, yes, I remember," her father said.

"Then let's proceed with the ceremony," his daughter said.

The young couple were married and the rich businessman gave them one of his apartments to live in.

One day passed.

Two days passed.

Three days passed.

But the girl didn't dare to give her new husband the seven blows. Her husband, too, was concerned. When was that day going to come? And what should I do about it?

The next day he was sitting in his meditation room. He saw his wife coming from a distance with a shoe in her hand. He happened to be reading the Bhagavad Gita, the verse were Krishna was telling Arjuna not to be a coward, that being a coward didn't fit his character.

His wife opened the door to his meditation room and entered. She was carrying a shoe and had a determined look on her face. It so happened that the family cat also came into the room when his wife opened the door. There was a sword hanging on the wall in the room. It had no purpose other than decoration. It was an old sword, but it was sharp, and just hanging there.

All of a sudden he got an idea. As soon as his wife approached him, he closed the door so neither his wife, nor the cat, could get out. Then he roared with great anger,

"YOU CAT!" And saying that, he pulled the sword from the wall and ran after the cat.

"YOU CAT!" He screamed again, in total rage. "IN MY MEDITATION ROOM!" And he gave one blow and cut the head off the cat.

His wife was horrified and dropped her shoe.

"AND YOU!" He screamed, turning to his wife, "C'MON! GIVE ME SEVEN BLOWS!"

His wife shook with fear. Then she fell down weakly at his feet.

"I will never hit you," she said tearfully.

"ARE YOU SURE!" He screamed.

"Yes, yes," she said. "I'll never beat you."

Then he calmed himself and lovingly told her to leave the room. He took care of the cat, and the sword, washed it and so on. In India they believe that if you kill a cat, you must give the equal weight in gold as a donation, and this he vowed to do.

"I'm going to the river for bathing," he gently told his wife.

He went to the river and truly prayed to God. I've done an awful thing by killing one of your creatures. Please forgive me, Lord, and he repented for his deed.

Days and days passed and his wife never remembered her shoe again. Then they lived happily.

What is the meaning of this story? We're married to our thoughts. Our destructive thoughts demand our attention, beating us on the head, causing us pain. If we want to get rid of them, we must do it with great firmness. We must cut them, with one blow of the sword, like cutting the head of the cat. Then only can we have peace.

STORY #9

There is such unusual power in love. When we express this love for God, we're also loving our family, our community, and our nation. Our life becomes full of joy and loving others becomes our nature. If we want to be happy, we must give this happiness to others. God is clever. He has planned things in such a way that our happiness is locked within others, and their happiness is locked within ourselves. The key that opens that lock is love. Love comes from the heart and it opens the heart of the other.

A FLOWER FOR LORD BUDDHA

ONE DAY LORD BUDDHA entered a town. He was famous by then and soon everyone had gathered for his darshan. There were of thousands of people.

Everyone brought him a flower because flowers are soft and gentle and he himself was the gentlest flower. So they picked all the flowers in the city and made garlands and brought these to Lord Buddha and put them around his neck and laid them at his feet.

That evening a poor gardener was walking through his small garden. Because the demand for flowers had gotten so high, he was carefully inspecting his flowers. He noticed one beautiful rose in the corner of the garden. It was blooming just at the right time and was exceptionally fragrant and stunning. He knew this flower would bring him lots of money.

Two rich men walked by.

"Look at that rose!" One of them said, and they walked over to the flower.

"Would you like to sell it?"

"Yes, that would be fine," the gardener said.

"How much do you want for it?"

"You tell me," the gardener said. He knew flowers were scarce in the city.

"I'll give you one gold coin for it," the man said.

"I'll give you ten!" the other man said.

"I'll give you one hundred!"

"I'll give you one thousand!"

The gardener thought he was dreaming. He was poor and money was scarce. No flower could be worth this much money. A whole garland of flowers would never be worth this much.

The men kept arguing.

"I'll give you ten thousand gold coins, my final offer! What do you say?"

The gardener thought for a moment and then he said to himself,

"If I can find out who this flower is for I could get even more money from that man. He must be fabulously rich."

"Who's the flower for?" He asked.

"We want to give it to Lord Buddha," the men said. "He's staying in our town."

The gardener had never heard of Lord Buddha. He had been too busy scratching out a living.

"I don't want to sell the flower," the gardener said. "I want to give this flower myself to Lord Buddha. Where's he staying?"

"Just follow the crowds," the men said with great disappointment. "They'll lead you to him."

The gardener carefully picked the fragrant rose. By now it was dusk and Lord Buddha had finished giving darshan for the day, so there were no crowds to follow.

"Where's Lord Buddha staying?" The gardener asked someone.

"Outside of town," the person said. "Follow that road."

The gardener found where Lord Buddha was staying for the night. The swamis who were serving Lord Buddha received him kindly.

"I have a flower for Lord Buddha," he said.

The swamis saw the beautiful rose, yet they couldn't disturb Lord Buddha. He had already begun his evening meditation. But they were kind-hearted and didn't want to disappoint this man who had walked so far.

"Lord Buddha is meditating," they said, "but come with us and you can see him from a distance."

They pointed to a big tree and there was Lord Buddha, meditating quietly under the tree.

When the gardener saw Lord Buddha he forgot all about his desire for money. He had come here to sell his rose to a rich man, but now that thought left him. Slowly he walked toward Lord Buddha and he bent down and placed his flower at Lord Buddha's feet. Lord Buddha was meditating with great peace and that peace filled the gardener's mind and body and spread into his heart.

At that moment Lord Buddha opened his eyes. His compassionate gaze fell upon the gardener and the flame of love burst into the gardener's heart and he bowed to Lord Buddha with tear-filled eyes.

"Truly this is a rich man," the gardener whispered. "I've received millions of gold coins from him, the gold coins of love."

STORY #10

Decisions should be made only under the calm condition of the sat-tva guna, or pure state of mind. This is where willpower resides. Decisions made from rajo guna, the excited state of mind, or from tamo guna, the state of lethargy, are weak and short-lived. The motivation which truly inspires us to do what's good for us, isn't something we can borrow from others. It must come from within us. Borrowed inspiration is short-lived and persists only in the presence of the motivator.

We each have this innate ability to inspire ourselves. The power of this inner inspiration is long-lived and motivates us continually along our chosen path. Obstacles may arise, but we overcome them. Genuine seekers are courageous warriors. They never take a step backwards. They are one-pointed: "Am I headed for this shore or not? What's my decision?" That's what they ask themselves everyday.

THE FARMER'S VOW

ONCE UPON A TIME a scholarly, nonattached saint traveled to a large city and stayed in a spiritual inn. Within a few days, the people had learned of his arrival. Many people gathered for his darshan, and a few scholars humbly asked him,

"Beloved Saint, we would love to hear your divine voice. Please grace us with the nectar of your speech."

The saint consented and gave a series of discourses. Enchanted by his pure speech, the people were saturated with love. Peace and gentleness filled the city. As a result, many people were inspired to perform spiritual practices.

A month passed, and eventually it was time for the saint to depart. The saint gave his farewell discourse and the people were sad.

"Now you will go somewhere else," they said. "We can't stand being separated from you."

The saint comforted them by saying,

"Only when we forget someone are we separated from them. When we continually remember someone, there is no separation. Remembering is part of the union between two people. Forgetting is part of the separation. If you wish to remember me, choose a vow to make. Then you will remember me each time you practice the vow, and your life will also be disciplined. Your will power will increase by observing your vow, and you will succeed at whatever you wish."

The people loved the idea. So, one by one, each person went up to the saint, bent close, and whispered their vow.

The first person said,

"I'm addicted to cigarettes. From now on, I won't smoke."

The second person said,

"I have a drinking problem. From now on, I won't drink."

The third person said,

"I argue with others too much. From now on, I'll speak less."

The fourth person said,

"I've never tithed. I'll tithe regularly from my earnings."

In this way, everyone made a vow they thought they could keep.

There was a farmer named, Govinda, in the crowd. He had come for ten days to hear the saint speak. He wasn't interested in spiritual growth, yet the saint had inspired him to make some changes in his life. He approached the saint humbly and bowed to him. Then he stood up quite worried and stammered,

"Mahatma, I'm not interested in the Lord, or devotion. Nor do I spend time away from my farm. I'm not able to observe a difficult vow. What should I do?"

"Take a vow you find easy," the saint replied with love.

"But I can't decide what vow to make. Please give me one simple discipline to practice."

"Very well," the saint said. "You should eat your meals only after you've seen someone's face."

"That's simple enough," Govinda said, quite satisfied. "Will any face do?"

"Yes. Who you see isn't important," the saint explained. "Your determination to observe the vow is important."

"I don't mind taking this vow, then," the farmer said. "So I vow that every day for a year and a quarter, I'll eat my meals only after looking at someone's face."

The saint blessed the farmer and the farmer left.

Once the farmer got home, however, he thought this over more carefully.

"How am I going to do this?" He said. "Shiva's temple is far from my house, so I can't go there every day. Krishna's temple is close, but they only give darshan at scheduled times, so that won't work. And I'm always hungry, just starved, after working in the fields all day. So if I choose a face, and can't find that face when I'm hungry, that would be awful. I'd better be careful about this."

Then Govinda saw the potter's house across the field. Every day the potter's donkey stood in the same place in the field. The donkey was there in the morning when Govinda set out for his fields, and he was there in the evening when Govinda returned to his house, always in the exact same spot. So, Govinda decided that he would eat only after seeing the donkey's face.

Three months passed.

Every day during this time, Govinda had glanced over at the donkey and seen his face before he had eaten, so he had kept his vow without any problem.

Then the monsoon season arrived. As usual, the farmwork increased and Govinda had a longer work day in the fields. One evening, after a long day of hard work, Govinda was famished. Driven by hunger, he walked quickly home. He glancing toward the potter's house, but that evening the donkey wasn't there!

He was terribly hungry and so he became angry at everyone... at himself and his foolishness for taking the vow, at the saint for inspiring him to take it, at the potter and his donkey who wasn't there now when he was hungry. So he decided to talk himself out of the vow.

"What good is this vow, anyway?" He said, driven by hunger.

But then determination returned.

"All my life I've never committed myself to any vow," he said. "This is my first chance, and it isn't right to break it."

He walked over to the potter's house. The potter's son was home and Govinda asked, "Where has Shamalbhai gone with his donkey?"

"My father and mother have gone over there, behind our house to get some sand," the son said, pointing in the direction of a nearby hill.

Wanting to find the donkey and keep his vow, Govinda hurried toward the hill, wiping perspiration from his face. In a short time, he reached the hill, but the donkey had his back to him. Since he had vowed to look at the donkey's face, he couldn't return after seeing only the donkey's tail, so he walked closer.

At that very moment, something extraordinary was happening to the potter and his wife. While digging in the sand, they had found a chest full of golden jewelry. The potter and wife were hugging themselves in ecstasy, just as Govinda arrived. Although they had looked around to make sure no one had seen them, they were now too jubilant to be watchful, and hadn't seen Govinda approach.

By the time they glanced up, they saw Govinda quickly walking away, and immediately became suspicious that he had seen the treasure and was running to tell the authorities.

"We must convince Govinda not to tell the authorities!" Shamal said quickly to his wife. "They'll take the whole fortune from us!" She agreed immediately.

"Govindabhai!" The potter yelled. "Wait a minute!"

Govinda glanced back, waited a moment, and then said,

"Yes, I've seen it," meaning the donkey's face.

The potter misunderstood, convinced that Govinda had seen the treasure.

"Govindabhai, dear neighbor," Shamal said in a sweet voice, "We know you've seen the treasure we dug up. But if you report this to the government, none of us will benefit from this wealth. It would be best to split the treasure between us and keep quiet."

Govinda had no idea what the potter was talking about, but he wisely remained silent. Without saying a word, he accompanied the potter back to the site of the treasure. Then he consented to his neighbor's proposal and split the treasure, firmly convinced that he had received this boon by practicing his simple vow.

Govinda wrapped his share of the treasure in a thick cloth and headed home. That night, he ate peacefully with a contented mind. His faith in the saint who had given him the vow had grown strong.

If we observe spiritual disciplines with determination, will we also discover buried treasure? Yes, if we maintain our determination, we will definitely find buried treasure, not from sand in the earth, but from the depths of the heart. Great masters often say, "The Beloved Lord lives in the palace of determination."

STORY #11

The Lord secretly nourishes the sun and the moon with light. He secretly fills the earth with food. He secretly fills the clouds with water. Yes, we can clearly see the sun, the moon, the light, the earth, the food, the clouds, and the water, but our eyes can't see the Lord, or any part of His body, or even His shadow. The Creator of the world is so great that He works in silence. Since we are His children, shouldn't our nature contain a bit of His charity?

The charity loved by the Lord has two wings: Give secretly, and, Give and forget. That is, as much as possible we should give without others knowing. Pure charity is only that which we give with compassion and religious feeling. When a devotee offers pure charity with faith to God and Guru, God and Guru feel tremendously content and merge with the devotee, making him or her Their own.

In The Name of Lord Buddha, I Have Received the Alms

ONCE UPON A TIME, as the sun rose in the east, a town gatekeeper opened the magnificent doors of a city. A Buddhist monk stood outside with a begging bowl in his hand. Walking softly, with eyes lowered humbly to the ground, the monk entered the city.

Lord Buddha was a prominent master during this period, and his life had a profound influence on the people in this area. The entire city was practicing the teachings of Lord Buddha. Whenever people heard His name, they bowed their head in reverence.

As the rising sun spread its light in all directions, the townsfolk bustled about their morning routines. The monk, meanwhile, walked down the streets, pleading in a humble voice,

"In the name of Lord Buddha, please give me alms."

No one could understand, however, why the monk said, "In the name of Lord Buddha." To them the words, "Please give me alms," would have been enough.

But this was not an ordinary monk. His very presence revealed his extraordinary nature. His steady gaze was focused on the ground, for he sought only alms, not wealthy people, so he looked only at the hands of his donors, not at their faces.

Everyone loved his voice. When he called, "In the name of Lord Buddha," it was full of sweet compassion. The people in the neighborhoods all returned to their homes to find a proper offering for him. When they found something suitable, they ran quickly outside to give it to the humble monk.

But whenever someone in the town offered the monk alms, he drew his begging bowl back and walked on. It was as if he had come to look at alms only, but not to receive them.

People all over the city stood in their courtyards ready to offer alms. Yet the monk walked past each person with no more than a glance at what they offered.

Finally everyone thought that the monk had come seeking some special alms. Yet no one could figure out what the alms might be, since the monk seemed disinterested in the food, clothing, money, and jewels offered to him.

As the daylight faded and the monk continued to accept no alms, the people were worried. Their elation at having his holy feet bless their city and turn it into a place of pilgrimage, now was fading, as they didn't know how best to serve him, and they were afraid the humble monk would leave. By nightfall, the whole town knew the story:

"A great monk is walking our streets begging alms, but he won't accept anyone's offering."

The entire town was concerned. People in every home on every street searched for something they could offer the monk that he might accept.

"Surely, the monk will accept this!" They thought.

But then......the humble monk would walk past their home. Eventually, he walked past every home on every street in the entire town and didn't accept a single thing from anyone. "In the name of Lord Buddha," he continued to ask in his sweet voice, "Please give me alms."

Finally his gentle, pleasing voice became dry and hoarse. Not once did he sit down to rest. Not once did he put a single morsel of food, or a single drop of water, into his mouth. As the sun set in the west, his feet were tired from constant walking and his begging bowl was still empty.

At last the monk approached the city gate again, the same one he had entered at sunrise, and left the city with a heavy heart. He entered the forest surrounding the city and continued repeating the same plea,

"In the name of Lord Buddha, please give me alms."

His voice had lost its strength and was only a sweet whisper.

But then?

His eyes lit like lightening flashes. His ears became alert. His tired legs filled with new strength. He thought he heard someone calling him. Yes, it was the voice of a woman.

"Monk," she said. "Please come this way."

He walked quickly toward the voice. But why am I hurrying, he thought? He had no answer to this question. He was simply listening to his heart, and his heart was saying,

"Monk, walk swiftly to receive special alms. These alms are only for fortunate souls. Donors of such alms rarely take birth in this world."

The monk walked up to a huge old tree and stopped. From inside the hollow of the tree, he heard gentle words, "Reverend monk, you have showered abundant grace upon me by coming here. Please accept my alms."

From within the hole came an emaciated hand holding a torn, ragged cloth.

Extending his begging bowl, the monk accepted her offering. Tears rolled from his eyes, as he uttered three times,

"In the name of Lord Buddha, I have received the alms. In the name of Lord Buddha, I have received the alms. In the name of Lord Buddha, I have received the alms."

Yes, these alms were as unique as the name of the blessed Lord Buddha. And who was the woman offering alms? She was a Buddhist monk who lived deep in the forest and never ventured into the city. Eating only forest fruits and roots and drinking only river water, she followed the path of yoga prescribed by Lord Buddha. She didn't own even a pot for water. Her only possession was the ragged cloth she wrapped around her body, and today she had offered even that last possession. She was uniquely charitable in giving of her own Atman.

We're deluded if we think hoarding brings happiness. But it's our nature to hoard, so we can't immediately give up everything and jump out of the hoarding stage. We must gradually give things up and take medium-sized steps in that direction.

STORY #12

Greatness has its permanent abode in humility and shallowness of pride. Humility is the landmark of knowledge, while pride is the landmark of ignorance. The idea that if one bows down he is insignificant, and that if one doesn't bow down, he is great, is false. The branches of a tree laden with fruit bow low. An older person bends down to pick up a child. A full vessel pours out so that an empty vessel may be filled.

THE PROUD CROW

IT WAS EVENING TIME. A crow was sitting on the branch of a tree in the woods, when he saw a flock of swans. The swans had stopped to rest under a nearby tree. In the rays of the setting sun, their white bodies were attractive, and their presence filled the evening with beauty.

The crow was black and didn't like the white color of the swans. Nor did he like the arrival of the newcomers. So he came down from his branch and strutted proudly toward the swans. Then he stood in front of them and stared at each swan from head to tail.

"Where did you all come from?" He asked in a haughty manner.

The older swans, looking at the crow's proud walk, his mannerless speech, and stupid behavior, were amused. Nevertheless, they didn't express this on their faces. The young swans, however, couldn't resist laughing, although they tried to hide it out of good manners.

One young swan, though, didn't like the arrogant behavior of the crow. The young swan went up to the crow and spoke to him, as if he were speaking for the group.

"Dear friend," he said. "We've come a long distance. Please join us."

"I'm fine right here!" the crow said, disregarding the invitation. "I only approached you because one single thought came to my mind as I saw all of you."

"What thought was that?" The young swan asked. "Please tell us. And thank you for the grace of your presence. We're grateful."

"I see that you all look white and beautiful," the crow said. "But can you fly?"

"Oh," the young swan replied softly, so softly that only the crow could hear him and not the older swans, "Your Highness. You must be a great teacher who gives flying lessons. I feel like this is an important day for me."

The foolish crow was extremely pleased to hear this.

"Dear, boy," the crow said proudly. "Your guess is correct."

"By the grace of blessed God, I'm fortunate to be in your presence, Gurudev," the swan replied. "If you would give me a short lesson in private, I would be very grateful."

The crow was delighted. Such an excellent disciple he had! He granted permission and they both met in private.

"Gurudev," the young swan said, "How many flying techniques do you know?"

"All of them," the crow said proudly.

"How many techniques are there?"

"Fifty two."

"Really? Fifty two? Are there that many?"

"Yes."

"Would you bless this curious child and show me a few?"

"Certainly. Watch me carefully."

The crow jumped up and flew a few feet into the air, and returned to his original spot. The second time, he jumped up, circled to his left, and returned again. The third time, he jumped up, circled to his right, and returned.

"Stop! Stop, Gurudev!" The swan begged. "Please stop! That's enough!"

The crow stopped and came near his disciple. The young swan greeted his Guru by bowing and taking the dust of his Guru's feet on his head.

"The techniques you have shown me are extremely compli-cated," the swan said. "I'm not able to absorb them. Indeed, your knowledge is limitless. I have one last request. Please show me your fastest flying technique."

"I will," the crow said, "And do you also wish to fly with me?"

"Yes, sir. I'll try."

"You'll be tired," the crow scolded. "Flying with me isn't child's play."

"Guruji, if I get tired, I'll ask you to slow down.

The crow agreed without hesitation.

The roaring ocean was close nearby. The young swan gestured to the crow to fly in that direction. The crow took off over the ocean, flying fast to tire his disciple. The young swan stayed be-hind intentionally.

"Are you tired yet?" The crow said after a bit. "I'll stop if necessary."

"No, sir," the swan replied. "I'm not tired. Please increase your flying speed."

Over and over, the crow asked the same question, and over and over the swan answered in the same manner. When they were far out to sea, the crow became exhausted. His body slipped lower and lower, closer to the water. Finally, it touched the surface of the ocean and the proud crow started to drown. The swan looked at the pitiful crow. Death awaited him.

"Dear, Guru," the young swan asked. "What are you doing? Is this the fifty-third way to fly?"

The haughty crow said nothing now. He was close to death and couldn't utter a single word. Finally, the young swan said,

"Guruji, I only know one technique for flying. I'll show you that now. Climb unto my back and hold onto my neck."

The crow grabbed the neck of the swan and the swan flew with such great speed that the crow became dizzy. When they reached shore, the dizzy crow opened his eyes and fell to the ground uncon-scious, but saved from death.

Wise men do not praise themselves. If others praise them, they are not carried away. Nor do they think of themselves as men of great wisdom. Pride means multiplication; that is, a proud person makes a show of being many more times virtuous than he really is. Humility means division; a humble person makes little of his virtues and demeans himself. A proud person is blind because he sees only himself. Humility has divine sight, as he sees only others.

Good men try to hide their virtues and bad men try to hide their vices, but neither virtue nor vice can be hidden long. How can one conceal the perfume of flowers in a beautiful garden, or the putrid smell of a rotten corpse in a ditch? One should admit one's faults and be rid of them. An individual who cannot do without praise is like a cripple who cannot walk without crutches.

STORY #13

All my life I've deeply contemplated the subject of celibacy or brahmacharya. Truly, this is the most important subject for the entire world. I have contemplated this subject for only 50 years, whereas the ancient sages of India contemplated it for thousands of years. Our current understanding of celibacy is different from the ancient concept of brahmacharya, and is superficial by comparison. Their knowledge transcends the limits of body, mind, and intellect and has entered the unapproachable realm of the soul.

Repression of sexual energy leads to perversion. Sublimation of sexual energy through yogic disciplines leads to immense spiritual power. Just as energy generated by steam or electricity can power machines which perform great tasks, the celibate yogi can also accomplish amazing tasks by conserving sexual energy.

To produce steam, water and fire are necessary. To produce spiritual power, pranayama and celibacy are necessary. Experiment with pranayama and celibacy under proper guidance for a year and a quarter and see for yourself.

THE SAINT AND THE PROSTITUTE

VASAVDATTA WAS A BEAUTIFUL prostitute. She entertained aristocrats at her magnificent residence or sometimes in their palatial homes.

One enchanting full moon night, Vasavdatta was engrossed in beautifying her body. She wore make-up, sensuous clothing, and jewelry. Finally, she adorned her hair with fragrant flowers and sprayed expensive perfume on her sari dress. Her house was filled with sweet fragrance.

When it was time to leave, she entered her courtyard, and walked to where her charioteer stood waiting in his chariot.

Feeling delighted, Vasavdatta seated herself in the chariot and directed the charioteer,

"Sumantra, there is a radiant full-moon tonight. Drive along the lakeshore so we can enjoy its natural beauty."

She had an appointment with a rich man tonight, and she was going as a beloved to an appointment made by a lover. Her heart was blooming like a thousand-petaled lotus. Her lover's home was on a secluded spot near the lake. But as they approached the lake, Vasavdatta's eyes came to rest upon a different man.

There sat a Buddhist monk, Upgupatta, meditating with closed eyes. Radiant with the splendor of celibacy, his body glistened in the moonlight. Vasavdatta had never seen such a beautiful sight. She completely forgot the lover she had originally set out to meet. Was he then truly her lover? No, she was a prostitute with innumerable lovers, each with eyes thirsty for beauty and passion. How could pure love reside there?

Vasavdatta halted the chariot close to the shore. Quietly getting out, she approached Upgupatta. Her jingling anklets caught his attention, and he opened his eyes. Although he beheld a celestial woman standing before him, Upgupatta was not influenced by her arrival or by her beauty. Vasavdatta peered into his crystal clear eyes which contained neither passion nor desire for beauty. Never in her life had she seen such a pure and wholesome gaze.

"He must be a saint," she thought. "His body and mind are pure. It's a great sin to look at him with passionate eyes."

Yet, this thought didn't remain in her mind for long. Vasavdatta had mastered the art of overwhelming her lovers with passion, but now she found herself helpless for the first time. Was the thirst for pure love awakened in her?

While drinking the nectar of his beauty, Vasavdatta found herself gently praying to him,

"Oh, Divine One," she whispered. "I've accidentally come upon your feet, and in a mere moment I've become yours. Kindly accept me. I humbly beg for your love."

Hearing her request, Upgupatta's eyes were filled with pure love. When he spoke, there was no anger in his voice.

"Divine lady," he said kindly, "Right now I'm meditating. Let me continue and tomorrow I'll come to your home."

"You'll come to my home?" Vasavdatta said, astonished.

"Of course," he replied.

"Your Holiness, do you know who I am?" Vasavdatta asked timidly.

"No, I don't know who you are."

"I'm Vasavdatta, a well-known prostitute in this city."

"Where do you live?" Upgupatta asked in an unconcerned voice.

"Near the Devkunj."

"All right, then, that's where I'll meet you," he said.

Vasavdatta continued to gaze at him for some time without blinking, and finally asked,

"Won't you hesitate to come there?"

"Where is there hesitancy in love?" Upgupatta replied firmly.

The word, love, struck her ears like the sweet strumming of a sitar

"Do you love me?" She asked, longing to hear the word again.

"A few moments ago, you begged me for love," Upgupatta said with sublime steadiness, and once again, Vasavdatta experienced a tender joy.

"I must go now," she said. "I don't want to disturb your meditation. I'll wait for you tomorrow at lunchtime."

With that, Upgupatta immediately closed his eyes and continued meditating. Meanwhile, Vasavdatta seated herself in her chariot and directed the charioteer to take her back home.

For years, Vasavdatta had been playing at love for money as a prostitute. But today the flame of pure love had been kindled of its own accord in the temple of her heart. Feeling no longer like a prostitute, Vasavdatta now felt more like a pure adolescent, mentally married to her chosen husband. She smiled radiantly, certain that her few moments of exquisite pure love had far surpassed her years spent in passionate pursuits.

The next day was exciting in every way. Vasavdatta carefully bathed and dressed herself in white clothing. Someone unfamiliar with her would have guessed that she was an ascetic from the forest visiting the city. She and her maidservant transforming her home, removing expensive sensual material from the dining room and replacing it with a modest carpet. Next, she went to the kitchen and prepared simple food. Although Vasavdatta had a treasury of golden china, she asked the servants to bring plantain leaves for dishes. How could man-made utensils compare with the sublime beauty of God's creation?

Vasavdatta finished all her arrangements and eagerly awaited Upgupatta in the courtyard. When he arrived, Vasavdatta affectionately welcomed him and invited him to dine. Neither spoke during the meal. Upgupatta's eyes were pleased at the sight of the external changes.

After sitting for some time, he finally excused himself, saying he had to leave.

"You're leaving?" She replied with fright.

"Yes," he stated. "I came only to offer alms of love. My purpose is finished. Now I must leave."

"So this is love?" She inquired insistently.

"Yes," he replied. "Whatever satisfies the body and mind with a mere drop is called love."

"Your Holiness! But I haven't received the satisfaction of which you speak," asserted Vasavdatta.

"That's due to your own lack of penance," replied Upgupatta. "One can't attain love without penance. Only after penance purifies the body and mind can the nectar of love be secreted. If a mere drop of poison can cause death, then a mere drop of nectar can imbue immortality."

"But Divine One!" She protested. "Not only do I belong to this mortal world, but I'm even more impure and unworthy than an ordinary woman. My only desire in this life is that you touch me once more."

Upgupatta stood motionless.

"Divine and fair lady," he said, closing his eyes for a moment. "I promise you that I will come one day to bless you with a touch. Your penance is to wait until that time. I give my solemn promise."

"I have faith in your word and will wait for you," she said humbly.

As Upgupatta left, Vasavdatta collapsed to the floor.

Years passed. Stricken with the dread disease of syphilis, Vasavdatta began to experience its torment. Her beauty was painfully transformed into ugliness daily as the disease ran its course. At the same time, an epidemic of plague struck the city. Vasavdatta also fell victim to its ravages, and along with others who had become infected, she was cast out of the city into a ditch.

One night, when the full moon spread its light upon her, the sleeping Vasavdatta awoke slowly and in great pain. Upon opening her eyes, she experienced great thirst, but couldn't get up. She was close to death. Still, she yearned for a few drops of water to wet her parched throat. Looking around, Vasavdatta saw there wasn't a living person to be found, no one to help her. Only a few dead plague-ridden bodies lay off in the distance. There was no one to quench the thirst of the woman who used to drink from a golden cup. Her eyes filled with tears. Her only desire was for water and there was nothing she could do.

Then she heard someone's footsteps. Slowly turning her head in the direction of the sound, Vasavdatta was filled with joy and surprise. Upgupatta was coming. Her distress ran off into the distance while immense joy came running to her side. Indeed, it was he! It was the same body, splendid with the light of celibacy, which she had seen on the lakeshore. Now he was here by her side, just as bright and magnificent as ever.

Silently he sat down.

In a barely audible voice, Vasavdatta whispered,

"You did come after all! I'm so happy. Now I'll die in peace."

As Upgupatta took her head in his lap, Vasavdatta cried out loudly,

"No! No! Please don't touch me. My sickness will infect your body!"

Indifferent to her plea, he took her head in his lap and said with utmost love,

"Fair lady, don't trouble yourself. I promised to give you happiness with my touch. I've come to fulfill that promise."

Vasavdatta's eyes clouded with tears. Innumerable times she had experienced sensual pleasure, but the happiness of this sensation was beyond comparison. This was the touch of God. Her body, which had once competed with the charm of the moon, was now riddled with syphilis. But here was a new sensation! Where anyone else would have been repulsed, Upgupatta was showering divine love upon her.

As soon as he lifted the vessel of water, she remembered that her throat was parched. She opened her mouth. Experiencing her thirst quenched, Vasavdatta fell into reverie:

"Are these drops of water or of love?"

It was the taste love. As Upgupatta's hand affectionately caressed her head. Vasavdatta was satisfied drinking the nectar of love.

In a few moments, Vasvdatta felt her mind descending into unknown depths. The dark shadow of death was approaching her. Attempting to fold her hands in prayer, she looked up at Upgupatta, and with eyes fading into the darkness, she said her final good by to him.

Pray daily to the Lord. Observe celibacy, moderate diet, and exercise. Slowly proceed on the pilgrimage of life, carrying the lamp of good conduct in one hand and the lamp of sexual restraint in the other.

STORY #14

Today is Father's Day in your country. It will be an unforgetable day in my life. I was extremely touched by the way you came up to me and offered me your pranams, on your knees. There was great humbleness in that. Your love was coming from the very depth of your being. Really, if you were six or seven years old, I would have picked you all up and placed you on my lap, just to hold you. If you can love everyone with the same love that you loved me today your life will be full of happiness. The scripture of love is very ancient. We can't start love at 7 in the morning, or 8 in the evening. We must hold it in our hearts all day long.

COME WITH ME TO THE HOME OF THE LORD

ONCE IN INDIA THERE was a great saint named, Narad. He was a rishi, a highly developed yogi. One day he was walking and he came to his favorite town. The Lord, Himself, lived in this beautiful place.

"Whenever I come here I feel so peaceful," he told everyone.

"Then why do you leave?" They asked him. "Why don't you stay?"

"I leave because I want to bring everyone here," Narad answered. "I want to tell everyone about this beautiful place. Come with me to the home of the Lord! This is what I want to tell everyone."

The Lord, Himself, overhead this conversation.

"Narad," the Lord said, "Go and tell everyone about my beautiful town. Bring them all here. We'll wait for you."

"I'll leave right away!" Narad said with great excitement. "But, Lord, your town is too small. I'll come with thousands of people! Make your town a little bigger first and then I'll go."

"Actually, my town is a little too big already," the Lord said. "But please, Narad, go and bring us more people. Bring us everyone and then I'll make it bigger."

"I'll be right back!" Narad said, standing up immediately, "With thousands!"

Narad picked up his tamboura, the instrument he played constantly, and left the beautiful town.

He walked until he came to a new town and then he called together a large group of people.

"Come with me to the home of the Lord!" He said. "It's beautiful! Come with me! I'll be leaving soon! Do you all want to come?"

"Yes! Yes!" The people answered, and Narad was pleased because it was a large group of people.

"Remember," the leaders of the town said. "You've promised to take us to the home of the Lord, right? Don't forget."

"I won't forget," Narad said.

The people all got together and decided on their departure day. When the day came, Narad was extremely pleased. There was a huge crowd of people. Narad chanted and played his tamboura and led everyone in prayer. Then they left.

On the way they came to a woods. As the great crowd entered the woods, golden coins fell from the top of the trees. Everyone got excited and stopped and got busy collecting the golden coins.

"Stop!" Narad said, but no one listened.

"Guruji," the leaders told him. "We're definitely going to join you, but we'll be just a little bit late."

"Alright," Narad said. "Those who want to collect golden coins, stay here. But I'm leaving. Those who want to come with me must continue now."

Now the large crowd was cut in half.

Narad continued walking and those that remained started talking among themselves.

"Narad is a great yogi," they said. "If we follow him we'll acquire yogic powers. And look, because of him golden coins fell from the trees. Surely if we continue with him even greater things will happen to us."

Soon diamonds fell from the sky.

The people became giddy with joy and rushed to collect as many diamonds as they could.

"You foolish people!" Narad said. "Let them be!"

But no one heard Narad. They were all too busy collecting diamonds.

Now only four people remained.

"Brothers," Narad said. "Come with me to the home of the Lord."

"No," they said. "Look at all these people, so busy collecting diamonds. They've forgotten about the Lord. If we go with you they'll forget about the Lord altogether. We'll stay and become their teachers."

How cunning, Narad thought. He knew their minds. They wanted to let everyone else collect the diamonds and then they would get the wealth from the people through donations as spiritual teachers.

Narad walked alone back to the home of the Lord. The Lord was standing at the beautiful gate to the city waiting for him. Narad was so tired he couldn't even raise his head to gaze at the Lord. The compassionate Lord greeted him and took his hand and gave him a seat in the palace.

"Narad?" The Lord said softly. "You were going to bring a large crowd. What happened?"

Narad burst into tears.

"I told everyone about You and Your beautiful home. I chanted and prayed and played my tamboura, but in the end nobody came with me. They all had a reason why they wanted to stay."

If we don't leave the attraction for worldly things, how can the love of the compassionate Lord be born in our hearts? When our heart is filled only with love for the Lord, then our progress back to His home will be quick. Our progress on the spiritual path is directly proportional to the love in our heart. On this Father's Day, I pray to the Lord that He, the Father of us all, may come into our hearts. As children, we may forget Him, but He doesn't forget us. He will always care for us. He will always be our support. I give you my blessings today as your spiritual father and grandfather. May the love of the Lord be born in us all.

STORY #15

A STORY OF FORGIVENESS

O NCE I GAVE A talk in a small town. The people loved the talk so much that they wouldn't let me leave, and I ended up staying and giving spiritual discourses there for two months.

A few weeks after I left, a man visited the town and he heard everyone talking about me. He didn't like swamis very much. He had had one or two bad experiences. But he was impressed after hearing the people talk about me, so he told a friend.

"The next time this saint comes, let me know. I would like to meet him and serve him."

About a year passed, and then I was able to visit the town again. The friend sent a letter to this man telling him of my planned visit. The man was pleased and made plans to come and see me.

It so happened that I was late. A kind conductor offered me a seat on a train and I accepted it. At the first stop everyone in our car got off except myself and one other man. He must have been lonely, because as we continued on, he moved closer and closer to me, until he was finally sitting next to me.

"Where are you from?" He asked, and I told him.

"Where are you going?" He asked, and I told him.

And then he got mad.

"You're a swami, aren't you!" He said. "And you don't work, do you! You just roam around and around!"

"Yes," I said. "That's exactly what I do."

"Why are you wasting your life like this?" He said. "Find a good saint and go and stay with him and serve him. Study, and make something of yourself. I'm on my way to meet a high saint who everyone loves. Come with me and maybe he will help you."

I didn't say anything.

The train reached the small town where I was going and I got off. The man got off, too. It was evening and I needed to cross a river to get to the town so I walked quickly. The man did, too. We came to the river and I gave the boat keeper my ticket.

"Oh, look!" The man said sarcastically. "He has a ticket! He's not traveling free!"

We both got on the small boat, and three or four people immediately bowed down to me. The man laughed and made fun of them. Indian people bow down to any swami and he was laughing at that.

Then he noticed that there was a large crowd on the other side of the river and he got quiet. He must have thought that the Mahatma was there already and he was giving darshan.

The boat came to the opposite shore and the whole town had gathered to meet me. Someone had told them in advance of my arrival, even though I was late. When everyone saw me they immediately started chanting and singing and 5 or 6 people rushed to carry me from the boat to the shore so my feet wouldn't touch the muddy water.

"No! No!" I begged, but it didn't make any difference. They picked me up and gently placed me on the shore and then everyone bowed down and touched my feet and offered me flowers.

The man was totally shocked. He just stood there. This was the same man who had been coming to see me. He, too, was late that day and we had met by chance. Then his friend called to him.

"Gopal!" His friend called. "You received my letter! And you've already had a chance to meet swami! How wonderful!"

The man burst into tears. He was ashamed of himself now. He touched my feet and said,

"Only you could bear such harsh words from me. I insulted you very much. Please forgive me."

I embraced the man and held him with love and he was happy.

STORY #16

Man, who lives in darkness, thinks 'Look at me! Look at all the things I'm doing!' Yet God is so great that He hides behind His creation. We should give thanks to Him and remember Him from whom we draw our strength.

THE STRAW ON THE RIVER GANGES

ONE DAY THE RIVER Ganges was flowing beautifully out of the high Himalayas. The sun was bright on the pure, clean water. There was a sudden gust of wind and the wind picked up a straw and dropped it on the current of the river.

"Look at me!" The straw said. "This river is so beautiful! I'm passing flowers and woods and I can see all the mountains and overhead the sky is blue!"

The river kept flowing and passed one holy place after another.

"Look at me!" The straw said. "I'm passing all the holy places of India."

They came to a place where a lady was gathering water by the side of the river. She had a bucket and she dipped her bucket into the river and the straw went into her bucket.

"Look at me!" The straw said. "This lady will carry me throughout the town. I've found the holy place meant for me."

"Good by, straw," the river Ganges said. "I'm going to keep going, but you stay here if you want. I've taken you to all the holy places and I'm pleased that you found a place that you like. But first, though, don't you think you should thank me?"

"Thank you?" The straw said. "For what?"

"For carrying you," the river said. "You floated in my current and I brought you here."

"No!" the straw said. "Didn't you see me swimming? I wasn't floating; I was swimming."

"Little straw," the river laughed. "You were floating, not swimming. You did nothing on your own. You didn't have the strength to swim on your own in my water and if you had, you would have swam all over the place and not arrived at this holy spot. Go now if you want to, live here and be happy, but give thanks to God."

And the river left.

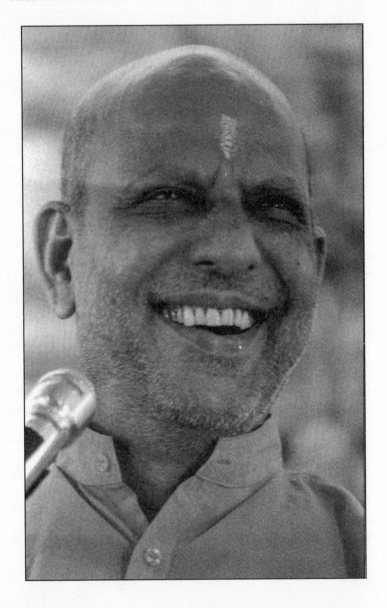

STORY #17

*If someone asked me, "Bapuji, can you accept insult and praise
equally?" I would reply, "No, I'm working toward it, but up to
now I haven't attained that stage." It's easy to study and teach
spiritual scripture, but to live a spiritual life is very difficult.*

LORD BUDDHA DEMONSTRATES THE DHARMIC LIFE

ONCE LORD BUDDHA WAS giving a sermon. A large crowd
had gathered for his darshan. When he was finished
speaking, the huge gathering slowly dispersed, except for
one man. The man was a religious opponent and drew close to
Lord Buddha, but he didn't bow down.

The loving, compassionate eyes of Lord Buddha quickly rested
on the man, but the man erupted into anger. His body trembled
and his eyes flared with animosity.

There wasn't the slightest disturbance in the heart of Lord
Buddha by this sight, nor was there any transformation in his
loving eyes. Perhaps the man felt that his anger would make an
impression on the mind of Lord Buddha and make him unsteady.
But when this didn't happen, the man became even angrier and
he stepped closer to the Buddha and spit in his face with great
hatred.

Lord Buddha's self respect wasn't wounded in the slightest
way by this bad conduct. He wiped the spit from his face with his
shoulder cloth and got up to leave for the monastery where he was
staying.

"Beloved brother," he told the man. "If you've finished your
statement may I go now to my residence?"

"My statement!" The man replied. "But I haven't spoken a
single word to you!"

"That's true," Lord Buddha said. "But you made your statement through your actions and I've listened carefully to your silent
statement."

The man said nothing and Lord Buddha left, assuming the encounter was over.

The man went home, but he couldn't sleep that night. The impression Lord Buddha had made on his mind was far deeper than he had received from reading any spiritual scripture. Reading scripture was ordinary. Today he had encountering the actual practice of the spirit of dharma.

The whole night the man lay awake. He analyzed his bad behavior and he was ashamed of himself. The dharmic actions of Lord Buddha had changed his heart.

The next day the man returned to the same place and listened to Lord Buddha's words again. But this time the man listened with a steady, loving mind and he pondered the words of Lord Buddha deeply.

When the crowd left, the man went up to Lord Buddha with downcast eyes. He put a garland of flowers at Lord Buddha's holy feet and cried for fifteen minutes unable to stop, looking with sorrowful eyes into Lord Buddha's gentle face.

Once again love flowed compassionately from the Buddha's eyes. He waited until the man was completely done crying and then he stood up and said,

"Beloved brother, if you've finished your statement may I go now to my residence?"

The man bowed down and touched the feet of Lord Buddha and whispered,

"Yes."

And he realized a great truth, that only a master can accept insult and praise with equanimity.

STORY #18

The Lord has said, "My devotee is greater than I." Who else but the compassionate Lord could say something so simple and loving? Likewise the noble saints have said, "The parents of a saint are greater than the saint." If the saint is the ocean, then his or her parents are the clouds. The greatness of the saint is evident, but the greatness of the parents is hidden. The higher greatness must conceal itself to make the lesser greatness look greater.

Noble saints in India after taking the vow of renunciation travel everywhere in society and they keep the same affectionate, selfless relationship with the world as a whole as they did with their original family. Sanatan Dharma, the eternal religion of India, prescribes that saints continually develop the feeling that 'The entire world is one family.' Thus, the renunciate cultivates a more expansive feeling of love for his world-family to which he subordinates his feelings of love for his original family.

The Day My Mother Became My Disciple

ONE TIME IN A village in India the members of the spiritual fellowship extended a special invitation to my mother and she stayed there happily for a few days. While returning home, she shyly said to me,

"Swamiji." She reverently called me swamiji because I had been initiated as a renunciate. "Now I'm old and can't follow you around wherever you go. If you come home to Dabhoi just one night a year, I'll be content."

I affectionately gave my consent.

About a year later I was on my way to Rajpipila. Suddenly I remembered the promise I had made to my mother as I approached Dabhoi, which was in the same direction. I walked home and it was lunchtime. My mother was performing her daily puja. She was overjoyed to see me, but continued her worship until she was finished.

Ten minutes later, carrying a ceremonial tray, she came gently toward where I was sitting. She sat down in front of me and I was surprised. I didn't know what she was going to do.

"Extend both of your feet," she said, in the sweet voice of a young girl.

"My feet?" I asked. I was sitting cross-legged in the chair. "Why?"

"I want to wash your feet. Today I want mantra initiation from you. I want you for my guru. I have great faith in you, for you have never deceived me. My husband was a devotee of the Lord and both of my sons are renunciates. Now, like a solitary tree standing in the desert, I'm all alone in this world. I want to pass the rest of my life in devotion to the Lord. Swamiji, please briefly give me guidance so that I'll die in peace. I've spent all these years without a guru, just to meet you, the Sadguru. I'm illiterate and foolish, but I have faith that you'll take me to the opposite shore."

Her throat was so choked with emotion that she could no longer speak. Although Mother had always tolerated pain well and rarely cried, she was crying profusely now. Each word had pierced my heart for I had never felt her speak so soulfully. During my youth, she generally spoke little and would mostly listen, since her husband and sons had dominant temperaments.

My eyes overflowed with tears and I stood up and embraced her. Now I saw her greatness and I realized that the mothers of the saints of ancient India must have been this simple, affectionate, and religion-loving.

I bowed down at her feet and sobbed,

"Mother, you've spoken so beautifully. But you're my guru! You shouldn't speak this way. You have inspired me, and you're the boat that takes everyone to the opposite shore. A boat doesn't need another boat. You don't need me to take your boat to the opposite shore."

My words had no impact on her at all.

"Do you still consider me to be your mother?" She asked, "Even after being initiated as a swami?"

"Of course," I said. "How could I forget to honor you as my mother? You're an extraordinarily special mother. You fed me, not just with your milk, but with liberation itself."

"Give me mantra initiation, then," she said firmly. "Just as you have initiated others." She had reached her final decision, so I sat back down. I knew the discussion was over.

Then she washed my feet with great love. After puja, I gave her mantra initiation with the proper guidance.

Finally, she reverently bowed down to me and offered me one and a quarter rupees as homage to her guru. Then she fed me the foods that I liked the most.

Whenever I remember this special event, I drown in the depths of my mother's greatness.

STORY #19

Service is the heavenly beauty of love. Service is the sweetest fragrance of love. Service is the bright light of love. Service makes one out of two, oneness out of duality. Service is the love process that makes two hearts beat as one, two souls or two lives as one. It begins with surrender and blooms into service and is the wealth of love. Service is the river of love. It purifies all.

THE WOMEN AND THEIR DEAREST TREASURE

ONCE IN A SMALL city in India fear was everywhere. The people were Hindu and a powerful Moslem king and his army had surrounded the city. The people were certain they would all be slaughtered. The army had appeared quickly with no warning, and there had been no time to get help elsewhere. They were totally outnumbered and at the mercy of the powerful king.

Perhaps the king would only demand money and wealth and then leave. This was their hope. This was at least tolerable because they could replace their wealth. But if he turned his army lose on the city with violence, rape, and death and demanded conversion, as well, then they would all suffer greatly.

The Moslem king knew the city was defenseless, that it had no army, that it was completely surrounded, and that no one could escape without his approval. Part of him wanted to plunder the city and reward his soldiers with whatever they wanted. But he wasn't an uneducated plunderer. He had been born into a royal family and he had been taught kindness, not cruelty and fanaticism.

So the king thought deeply about what to do. Then he made his decision. He would allow his men to rob the city of all its wealth, but harm no one, especially the women. Moreover, he would allow the women to leave with one bundle on their heads, carrying anything they wanted to save before his army entered the city.

They could save jewelry, costly items, expensive clothes, family treasures, whatever they wanted, but only one bundle.

The king then sent his messengers into the city with the news.

"The women may leave!" The messengers announced. "But they must be gone by 8 a.m. tomorrow morning! And they may carry one bundle on their heads with anything they want to save! Then our army will enter the city and take what we like!"

At 6 a.m. the next morning, the procession started, thousands of women left the city carrying one bundle on their heads. They were fearless because the king was true to his word. He had unblocked the main road out of the city and was allowing the women to leave unmolested as he had promised.

The king, himself, watched the procession. But soon he was puzzled. All the women, young and old, even grandmothers, carried one huge bundle on their heads. The bundle weighed so much that their legs wobbled and they could scarcely walk far without resting.

"How can gold, jewelry, and precious items weigh so much?" The king thought to himself. "What are these women carrying, anyway, that's so heavy? I'd better look into this. Maybe it's a unique treasure found only in this area of the world."

"Everyone stop!" The king commanded. "Stop walking and put your bundles down!"

The women followed the king's order helplessly. They were terrified and certain that now the king would go against his word and harm them.

"Untie each bundle!" The king commanded and everyone willingly obeyed.

The king was astonished! There were no jewels, gold, silver, diamonds, money, pearls, expensive cloths, or costly items in any of the bundles. All of the women had left these things back in their homes for the soldiers to take. They had no attachment to these things.

What then was in the bundles?

There were children and old men and husbands and brothers and sons.

The king laughed.

"Are these your most expensive possessions?"

The women all remained silent. No one dared to answer the king. Then an old woman spoke who cared nothing for her life anymore.

"Oh, great king," she said. "The dharma in which we were raised taught us to love and serve our husbands, our children, our parents, and our grandparents. We regard them as our most price-less possessions. They are the all-in-all in our lives. They are our wealth, our gold, silver, diamonds, and pearls. We believe them to be Parabrahma, Almighty God, the dharma, the truth, and Holy place of pilgrimage. We are simply practicing our heavenly dharma, the true dharma of our womanhood."

This plunged the king into deep thought. How could he plunder these people, where such love and service existed among them? He turned away completely satisfied and returned to his country with his army without any act of aggression upon the helpless city.

Story #20

*The Lord is the giver of the fruits of our actions and He is just.
He's always on the side of truth. And so we should try to make
good decisions with planning and proper understanding and then be
satisfied and forget about it and understand the laws of karma. If
we bring unhappiness and pain to others, we'll receive unhappiness
and pain in return. A farmer can't sow wheat and harvest corn.
Whatever the Lord does is always in the best interests of everyone
concerned.*

The King and His God-Loving Minister

ONCE THERE WAS A king. He had a God-loving, devoted
minister. No matter what happened in the kingdom,
good or bad, the minister would always say,
"Thy will be done, Oh, Lord."
The king thought this was foolish, but he put up with it.
One day the king was chewing on a piece of sugar cane and he
accidentally cut his finger and it started bleeding.
"Thy will be done, Oh, Lord," the minister said, looking at the
bleeding finger of the king. "God must have done this for some
reason."
The king got angry.
"What are you babbling about?" He shouted. "I cut myself
and it hurts! How can this be good for anything? Guards! Get this
stupid man out of my sight! Lock him up!"
A few days later the king was hunting. It was his favorite
pastime. Normally he would take his minister with him, but the
minister was still in jail, so this time he took other attendants.
They spotted a deer and the chase began. But the other attendants didn't know the area as well as the minister and soon they
were lost. Then they became separated and the king was suddenly
alone in the forest.

There were tribal people living in that part of the forest and they believed in human sacrifice. They were looking for someone to sacrifice to their gods and they captured the king riding alone on his horse.

They took him to their temple and their high priest was pleased. Here was someone dressed in fancy clothes and riding a beautiful horse, certainly a perfect sacrifice. The king begged for his life, but they only laughed and strapped him to a stone table. The high priest raised a sharp knife to cut off the king's head and then someone shouted,

"Wait! Look at his finger!"

These people had one condition for a human sacrifice: the person couldn't have any wound or defect on his or her body; they had to be perfect or their gods would be angry.

"Let him go!" The high priest said with disgust, putting his knife down. "He won't due."

The king quickly left on his horse, greatly relieved, and now he believed his God-loving minister, for certainly the king would have died a terrible death that day had it not been for his cut finger.

"Release the minister!" the king ordered when he returned home, "And bring him to me."

The king told the entire incident to the minister and then the king said,

"Now I believe you. Everything happens by the will of God. But I have one question for you."

"Yes?" The minister said.

"Because of my wound, I was saved a terrible death. I understand that. But what possible good came from me throwing you into jail so unjustly?"

"My king," the minister answered. "Every time you go hunting, you always take me with you. I have no wound on my body, and if you had taken me along they certainly would have sacrificed me!"

STORY #21

It's best to grow slowly but steadily on the spiritual path. Our progress is directly proportional to our love for the goal, because only love can create the necessary strength or power to progress. The seeker must acquire many spiritual qualities. If we try to obtain them all at once, we'll fail. One by one, we should try. Getting rid of a bad character trait is just as good as acquiring a new one. When we travel from one place to another, we naturally separate ourselves from the old place as we approach the new place. With great patience and self-forgiveness we should continue on and not be fooled along the way.

THE FAN THAT LASTS A HUNDRED YEARS

SUMMERTIME IN INDIA IS extremely hot. One day a man was selling his fans. The other fan dealers were selling their fans cheaper, but this man didn't care. He kept his price much higher.

As he slowly made his way through the streets selling fans, he came to the king's palace.

"Fans!" He called out. "Get the best fans in all of India! They'll last a hundred years! You may die, but your fan won't!"

The king heard this and was surprised.

"What kind of a fan would last a hundred years?" The puzzled king asked his servants. "Bring that fan seller to me."

The servants did as they were told and found the vendor. The fan seller was pleased the king was interested in his fans and he approached the king and paid his proper respects.

"Sit next to me," the king commanded. "Tell me about your fans. Do they really last a hundred years?"

"Yes, sir!" The vendor said with enthusiasm. "Guaranteed!"

"Show me these fans," The king said.

The vendor took out a few fans and showed them to the king. The king was disappointed.

"These are ordinary fans," he said. "They won't last 15 days."

"No," the vendor said. "They'll last a hundred years. Guaranteed."

"Are you sure of that?"

"Yes, sir."

"How much do they cost?"

"A hundred dollars each."

"A hundred dollars!" The king said. "They aren't worth ten cents!"

"Buy one and try it," the vendor said. "What I'm saying is absolutely true. I'll come back anytime you want and see how you're doing."

"Buy one of these fans," the king commanded his servants, "And show this man out of the castle."

Since it was a hot summer day, the king started using the fan right away. Normally, he didn't fan himself; he had servants who did that for him. But he was interested in this new fan, so he fanned himself with it.

The fan was completely destroyed in ten days.

"Bring that vendor back to me!" The king ordered.

The servants found the vendor out on the streets still shouting and selling his fans at a higher price, still claiming they would last a hundred years.

"Look at this fan!" The king shouted when the vendor returned. "It's totally ruined after 10 days and you said it would last a hundred years!"

"Perhaps you don't know how to use it," the vendor said.

The king thought for a moment.

"No, maybe not," he said. "How do you use it?"

"Here," the fan seller said, handing the king a new fan. "Let me see you fan yourself."

The king took the fan and started fanning himself.

"No! No! Not that way!" The fan seller said, taking the fan back. "Like this. Hold the fan very still in your hand and shake your head back and forth and the fan will last a hundred years."

If we are foolish like this, we'll never progress. Experiments with spiritual growth should be done properly.

STORY 22

Often the great saints say, "God is everywhere!" But if God is everywhere, why can't we see Him? We have eyes. Then why can't we see God if He's everywhere? This is an unusual situation. It's like a fish swimming in the ocean and yet asking, "Oh great water, where are you?" There are two reasons for not finding something: One reason is that we've forgotten where we placed it. The other reason is that even though the thing is right in front of us, we don't have the ability to see it.

THE DEVOTEE WHO COULDN'T FIND RAM

ONCE THERE WAS A devotee who searched everywhere to find Lord Ram. He cried and prayed to Lord Ram every day,

"Lord, Ram, where are you? Where are you? I want to see you. Please give me your darshan so that I may be happy."

The devotee met a saint and the saint told him,

"Lord Ram is in your heart. That's where you will find him."

The devotee was pleased. He sat under a tree and closed his eyes. He looked into his heart, but he didn't see Ram. Instead he saw great beasts with awful eyes and sharp teeth. These were the beasts of lust, anger, desire, jealousy, and fear, and they were trying to eat him. He was afraid of them and quickly opened his eyes and left.

The next day he cried and prayed to Lord Ram again.

"Lord, Ram, where are you? Where are you? I want to see you. Please give me your darshan so that I may be happy."

He met a second saint.

"I'm looking for Lord Ram," the devotee said. "Do you know his address?"

"Yes," the saint replied. "He lives in satsanga."

The devotee was pleased. Now he had Lord Ram's address. He attended satsanga faithfully over and over, convinced he would finally see Lord Ram. Yet, he never saw Lord Ram in satsanga, not even once.

So he cried and prayed again,

"Lord, Ram, where are you? Where are you? I want to see you. Please give me your darshan so that I may be happy."

He met a third saint.

"Kind, sir," the devotee asked, tired of his search now. "I'm looking for Lord Ram. I have faithfully followed the instructions of two saints, but I haven't seen Lord Ram."

"You can't see Lord Ram because your eyes are bad," the saint said. "You need glasses."

"Is there an optician nearby?" The devotee asked. "Where can I buy the glasses I need?"

"You can only buy the glasses you need from a Guru," the saint said. "And you have to pay for them and the price is expensive."

"What is the price?" The devotee asked.

"Pure character," the saint replied. "The first saint you met was correct. Ram is in your heart, but He sits behind the beasts of lust, anger, and greed. You must fight these demons. You can't be afraid of them and run away. You must remove them from your heart and then you will see Ram. The second saint was also correct. Ram lives in satsanga. But your mind must be peaceful. You must remove the pain, guilt, and sin from your mind and then you will see Ram."

We are all like that sometimes. Yes, God is everywhere, but we can't see Him because our eyes are bad. We must step firmly upon the spiritual path and battle our own demons with great determination and prayer and develop pure character. Pure character will bring purity to our heart, mind, and body and then we will see God.

STORY #23

When Devotion is still a little girl, she regards the ways of attaining God as toys and plays with them. When she attains maturity, she regards the means of attaining God as her greatest wealth.
Only then can she give birth to a child in the form of Knowledge.
When Knowledge reaches youth, Devotion then gives birth to a second child named Asceticism. The elder brother, Knowledge, is very fond of his little brother, Asceticism. The younger brother loves his elder brother to distraction. He cannot bear a moment's separation from his elder brother. Once Asceticism attains maturity, the Lord comes forth. Upon seeing Knowledge, Asceticism, and Devotion, the Lord becomes crazy with love.

THE KING AND HIS YOUNGEST QUEEN

ONCE UPON A TIME, a King had seven queens. Of all his queens, he loved the youngest one the most. She served him obediently, treasured his happiness, and was never unhappy.

The other queens tried to control the King. When the King visited, they often fought with him, or among themselves, and were cheerless. The King would leave with a deep wound in his heart. But when he visited his youngest queen, he would lose all concerns for affairs of state. Her loving, cheerful heart would soothe his troubled mind.

One day, the King needed to travel abroad for six months. It took his attendants several weeks just to make the preparations. He instructed each queen to prepare a list of everything she wanted him to bring back from his trip. The six unhappy queens prepared long, elaborate lists. Again and again, they reminded him,

"Now make sure that you get everything on this list, and take good care of everything in transit so that nothing is lost, broken, or spoiled."

The King reassured them that all would go well.

On the day of his departure, the King bid the six older queens farewell. He saved his final farewell for his favorite.

"Devi," he said gently, "You haven't given me your list. Please give me your list."

Following her husband's instruction, the youngest queen scribbled something quickly on a piece of paper and silently gave it to the King. Then she performed his puja with great love and tearfully bid him farewell.

"Come home soon in good health," she sobbed, choking on her words. "May the Lord protect you."

The King's eyes also streamed with tears, and he gazed at her with a heavy heart. None of the other six queens had cried while bidding farewell to him. In fact, their concern was only for the many gifts he would bring upon his return.

The King finally left, reluctant to part from the person who had captivated his heart.

He remained abroad six months.

As he made preparations to return home, he reviewed the lists from the seven queens. The six unhappy queens had written long lists of countless objects. The youngest queen, however, had written nothing except a large number, 'One,' on her list. The King couldn't imagine what this meant. He bought everything the other six queens had requested and then, still perplexed, carefully selected things he thought the youngest queen would like. Then he returned home.

Upon his arrival, the King visited the apartments of the six older queens. Predictably, each one gave him a shallow welcome, and then asked for their gifts. Their source of joy was the getting of gifts, and they inspected everything carefully. When the King went to the youngest queen's residence, however, she welcomed him with joyful eyes, bowed down to him, arranged for his bath and meals, and then finally asked how he was feeling. Her loving behavior touched the King's heart.

That evening, as the King relaxed in her presence, he remembered that the queen had written only the number, 'One,' on her list. Since he didn't understand what it meant, he was certain he hadn't been able to fulfill her request. He was pained to think that he might not have brought back her heart's desire.

"Devi," he said gently. "Your list just showed the number, 'One,' with no explanation of what it meant. I thought about it many times, but I couldn't figure out what you wanted. I feel sad that I wasn't able to bring you back the one thing you wanted. Unlike the others, you just wanted one gift, and I couldn't get it for you. Will you forgive me?"

"My Lord," she whispered sweetly, "You needn't ask for my pardon, because you haven't offended me. I've already received the, 'One,' that I asked for on my list."

"What do you mean?" The King asked perplexed. "I only brought you things that I liked. I'm delighted that you like them, too, but do they include the, 'One,' that you requested?"

"Yes, My Lord," the queen answered. "When I wrote the number 'One' on my list, I meant 'You.' I need nothing else. I only wanted my number 'One,''You.' And since you've come back from your journey fit and healthy, I've gotten what I had asked for."

Touched and pleased by her loving words, the King showered all the love he had in his heart on the Queen.

It isn't proper to act like the six older queens, and give the Lord a daily list of our demands: "Give me this. Give me that." And if He doesn't fulfill our demands, to act offended. True devotees of the Lord write only the number, One, on their list and place it before the Blessed Lord. All they want is God. They don't grieve and complain if God doesn't give them material things like food, clothes, wealth, house, and friends. Neither do they care if the Lord snatches away the material things they once had. They accept everything that comes into their life as His grace.

STORY #24

To donate one's time and energy can be a form of pure charity. Just as a morsel which drops from an elephant's mouth can feed millions of ants, a bit of time or energy donated to charity by a powerful person can alleviate the pain of countless people. Since our world is the Lord Himself, and the Lord is our world, serving any individual is as good as serving the Lord Himself.

THE BLIND BOY AND THE MUSICIAN

ONCE UPON A TIME, there were countless poor people living in huts on the outskirts of a large city. A middle-aged woman suffering from a disease lived in one of the huts. She was so emaciated and weak, that she couldn't sit up or move from side to side. Her husband had died the previous year, leaving her with a fourteen-year-old blind son and a twelve-year-old daughter.

Before her illness, she used to go to the city and perform hard labor. Her son and daughter used to go to the city, also. The boy would sit on street corners and play his small sitar and sing the bhajans of famous saints such as Kabir, Tulsidas, Soordas, and Meera. His voice was sweet, and people walking by would throw a few pennies, or a nickel, on a cloth he had spread on the sidewalk.

The earnings of the mother and son were meager, but the money was enough to cover their household expenses. They were all quite happy. The mother was disappointed by just one thing: she approved of her son singing bhajans, but she didn't like people regarding him as just a blind beggar boy, merely someone to toss a penny to. She believed in her heart that her son's income was what he earned as a musician, not as a beggar.

Then the bright days of happiness passed, and the dark days of misery descended upon the family. The mother became critically ill. Both children served their mother lovingly, but soon the food stored in their hut was gone. The mother needed to have one child remain at home to care for her. However, the blind boy couldn't go to the city alone. Yet if both children stayed home, how could the family possibly earn a living?

For two days, the children lived on just water, and they were able to provide a little food for their mother. Neither of the children felt the slightest hunger, nor did they even remember not eating. Their sole desire was for their mother to become well, and they did everything possible to bring this about.

One day, a generous doctor who selflessly served the poor, visited the family. He diagnosed the mother's illness and comforted the children by saying,

"Dear children, don't worry. Your mother is merely suffering from a fever, which is subsiding now. Her body is weak, but she'll be better within a week. Give her some orange juice if you can."

The children cried joyful tears. Even though they didn't have a crumb to eat, or a penny to spend, they were happy again. They borrowed money for orange juice and decided to go back to the city so they could repay the debt. Before they left for the city, they sat by their mother's side. She put one hand on each child and caressed them affectionately.

"I feel much stronger now," she said. "Run along to the city. I'll stay in bed. I'll pray to the Lord while you're gone."

Both children stood up. Although neither child had eaten for two days, they were both alert and joyful because their mother was stronger. The blind son took his sitar in his right hand, while his sister held his left hand. Then they left for the city with happy steps.

When they reached the city, the sister noticed a section of town that was more crowded than usual.

"Brother," she said. "This spot is the most crowded. Sit here and I'll spread the cloth. First though, pray to the Lord in your heart before beginning the bhajan."

By chance, a famous sitar player, one of the nation's best, was standing on the same corner. He had parked his car some distance away and was waiting for someone. The old, worn sitar in the blind boy's hand had caught his attention.

He watched as the small boy sat down and he overheard the sister asking her brother to pray before playing. Then he overheard the brother's response.

"Sister," the blind boy said, "As we were leaving this morning, mother said that she would be in bed praying to the Lord. I'm going to pray to the Lord, too, before beginning my bhajan. Will you also pray with me? I know that the compassionate Lord will hear our prayer. Our mother has a fever and hasn't had enough to eat for several days. If we get a little money today, we can bring her twelve oranges. I want to buy some food for you, too, since you've had only water for two days. You're younger than me, and younger children get hungrier than older ones. I don't feel hungry at all, and can continue for another two or three days on water. People who sing to the Lord never feel hungry."

The famous sitarist was overwhelmed and his eyes flooded with tears. He opened his wallet and removed a hundred-rupee bill, but then he thought for a moment, and put the money back. He moved closer to the children, hoping to hear more of their conversation.

The boy prayed silently for a moment. Then he played the prelude to a bhajan on his small sitar. Then he sang, Nath, Kaisegaja Ko Bandha Chhudayo, in a sweet voice full of pain and suffering.

Soon a small crowd gathered. Although the boy was too young to understand the deeper meaning of the bhajan, each word he sang was heart touching, as if his own tragedy were embodied in the tragedy of the poem.

The famous sitarist heard a future great singer in the boy's voice, and a future great musician in the boy's playing.

"How many pennies have we received?" the boy asked his sister, when he was finished with the bhajan.

"Only three or four," his sister replied in a worried voice.

"I hope we get more," the boy sighed.

"You've played only one bhajan," his sister said encouragingly. "Let's not worry. There's a big crowd today. I'm sure we'll get more money."

Her faith comforted her brother and enthusiasm returned to his heart. He sang another bhajan, Raghu Vir. Tumako Meri Laga.

When he heard the pitter-patter of coins falling on the cloth, he felt the Lord was helping them during this difficult time. In gratitude, he descended deeper into the feelings of the bhajan.

People came and went. The size of the crowd would dwindle and then grow again. By the end of the third bhajan, about one hundred listeners had gathered around the blind boy.

"We must have two rupees by now," his sister softly whispered into his ear.

The boy's eyes filled with joyful tears, which he quickly wiped away. He knew they could now buy oranges for his mother and food for his sister.

Just as the blind boy was about to begin his next bhajan, the famous sitarist approached him.

"Son," he said, gently and with affection. "Please give me your sitar. I'm curious to see how it plays."

Since the gentleman was dressed in expensive clothes, the sister guessed he was wealthy. "Give him your sitar, "she whispered to her brother.

The boy gave his sitar to the gentleman. The man sat down cross-legged on the ground and re-tuned it. Then he played, and when he played, the air was filled with sweet music. The beautiful strumming rejuvenated the aged sitar and within moments, a large crowd had gathered. Someone tossed a ten-rupee bill on the cloth. Another person tossed a five-rupee bill. Another person tossed a one-rupee bill. Soon money showered down on the cloth like rain.

The joy of the children was boundless! The blind boy, who loved music so much, had never heard such extraordinary sitar playing in his brief life. He couldn't see the gentleman, so he reached out and affectionately touched the sitarist, who patted the boy lovingly as he played.

As the sister watched this silent exchange of affection, her face bloomed like a thousand-petaled lotus. What a sight to behold!

Meanwhile, many listeners in the audience recognized the famous sitar player and guessed his charitable intention in playing this street-corner benefit concert. They were thrilled to listen free of charge to a performance that normally would have required expensive tickets a month in advance.

After playing the sitar for half an hour, the musician laid it in the child's lap and bowed to the audience.

"Friends," he said. "I sincerely thank you for listening to my music. I'm truly grateful to you all. I've performed many concerts in my day, but I've never experienced the joy I've received from today's performance. This is my lucky day. Truly, the Lord has showered abundant grace upon me, and I bow at His holy feet with faith and devotion."

As the people dispersed, the sister gazed in awe at the number of bills on the cloth. The artist picked up the money and placed it in her hand.

"Daughter," he said. "All this money is yours. I played the sitar for you alone."

"This is so much money," replied the sister. "And we live in a hut. What if someone steals it?"

"I'll deposit this money in the bank where it will be safe," the sitarist said. "Now let's buy some oranges for your mother and some food for both of you. Come, sit in my car, and I'll take you home after we buy the food."

Tears of joy rolled from the eyes of the children.

"You are gracious," they said in unison, "and we feel such love for you."

The musician experienced divine joy from their loving words.

They bought what they needed from the market and rode home to their hut in the sitarist's car. The mother was dumbfounded to see her children entering their hut with a rich gentleman who was carrying heaps of oranges and various foods. She couldn't comprehend what was happening. Joyfully the children told her their story. Over and over they glanced with affectionate eyes at the generous sitarist.

After hearing the whole story, the mother spoke in a voice choked with gratitude.

"Brother, you've done this poor family a great favor. How can I express my gratitude?"

"Sister," the famous sitarist replied meekly, "I accept your gratitude, but I haven't come to hear appreciation. I've come to share a few words with you about your son. He has a sweet voice, and I detect great potential in his playing ability. With your consent, I would like to return in a few days and take him to live with me. I'm an artist, and I want to train him to become an artist, too. We collected about 500 rupees today in our street-corner benefit concert. I'll deposit the money in a bank account under your name, and will also send you a little money every month for your living expenses. Within a few years, your son will become a great musician and you'll be able to live your life happily. In the meantime, feel free to visit your son at my home, and I'll also bring him here frequently to visit you."

The poor woman couldn't determine whether she was dreaming or awake. Eventually, she realized that she was awake and that this was all real. As tears streamed from her eyes, she murmured in a choked voice, "Brother, we're fortunate that you intend to make my blind son a great musician. I consider it an honor, so I don't have the slightest objection. As soon as I recover from my illness, I'll be able to earn a living easily for my daughter and myself. In the meantime, I'll gratefully accept whatever support you offer as being God's grace. My children and I have been praying to the Lord with a sincere heart for days. I feel that this truly expresses the miraculous power of prayer."

Then the mother fell silent, unable to utter another word.

STORY #25

*Sometimes only God can remove our faults. We're too weak on
our own. Then we should pray to Him: "My Lord, You're the
destroyer of all the demons. Let Your grace fall upon me. Hold my
hand and take me to Your lotus feet."*

LORD, CAST YOUR SWEET GAZE ON ME

ONCE A SAINT CAME to a town in India.
"My brothers and sister," he said. "Anger is a demon. Don't be angry with each other. When this demon
enters your mind, it creates pain and suffering in others. Give up
your anger."

A certain man was in the audience and he was moved by this
discourse.

"I'll give up anger!" He said to himself with great conviction.
"I will do this!"

He walked up to the saint afterwards and said,

"Your message went deep into my heart. I won't be angry
anymore!"

The saint wasn't impressed. He knew such a vow was impossible and yet he didn't want to discourage the man, either. So he
gently raised his hand and blessed the man.

"Yes, but do it gradually," the saint said. "Little by little, let
go of your anger."

"What do you mean?" The man said. "Why should I do it
slowly? I'll just push it out and be rid of it!"

"Yes, do that, then," the saint said, remaining calm. "Just push
it out and be rid of it."

"I will!" the man said. "I'm finished with anger!"

The man left and went home.

When he got home his wife had left a bowl of milk in the middle of the floor and the man stepped on it by mistake and spilled it.
Immediately, he got angry.

"Where are you?" He shouted to his wife.

His wife came running into the room and saw the spilled milk.

"Why did you leave this milk here?" The man demanded.

"I was getting some milk and the baby fell out of the crib," she said. "She cried, so I left the milk right there and ran to take care of the baby."

Now the man felt ashamed.

"I just promised that saint I wouldn't be angry anymore," he said, "And here I am angry already. And over nothing, too."

So he repeated his vow all over again, with even greater conviction:

"Anger is a demon! I won't be angry anymore!"

Then he thought,

"Now, how can I remember that? I know. I'll make a sign."

So he made a sign for himself with big letters that said:

One Should Not Be Angry. Anger Is A Demon.

He wrote the words on a board and put the board on his desk at work. Now he was happy.

But later that day he started arguing with someone at work and he got so angry he hit the man with the board.

Sometimes only God can remove our faults and we should pray to Him: "My Lord, cast your sweet gaze upon me. Come and take your seat upon the throne of my heart and smile and remove all my pains."

STORY #26

In traditional Indian society a true son or daughter serves their parents in their old age. Sanatana Dharma teaches that mother is divine and father is divine. There's one story in India about a great devotee who took this teaching to heart.

SHAMAN AND THE FLOWERS

ONCE THERE WAS A young man named, Shaman. A saint came to his town and Shaman heard the saint say, "Serve your parents. Consider your mother and father to be divine."

Shaman truly took these words to heart and he left that day determined to serve his parents.

Both of his parents were blind. So with great love he took over their daily routines. He got them up, gave them a bath, cooked for them, cleaned their house, washed their clothes, and took them outside for walks.

He did this with love and joy for two years.

Then one day his friends said,

"It's wonderful that you love your parents so much, but you should marry soon and have your own family."

Shaman thought deeply about this.

"What if I marry and my wife doesn't like this arrangement?" He said to himself. "Then everyone will be unhappy: my wife, my parents, and myself. It's best if I stay single and just serve my parents. They're blind and helpless."

So the years went by and his parents grew old and Shaman loved and served them and took care of their needs so they didn't suffer. When his parents were old, they desired to make a spiritual pilgrimage before they died. This was the custom, for elderly parents to make a spiritual pilgrimage once in their old age so their feet could touch holy ground and they could die in peace.

Today the pilgrimages are simple with roads and cars and airplanes, but in Shaman's day they had to walk and such a pilgrimage was difficult and dangerous. When a family in the village said they were leaving on a pilgrimage, the whole village gathered to say goodbye, not knowing if they would ever see the family again.

So on the auspicious day of departure, everyone gathered to say goodbye to Shaman and his parents and they all wondered the same thing: how was Shaman going to do this? His parents were blind.

And Shaman's mother asked, too,

"My son," she asked. "How are we going to travel?"

"Don't worry," Shaman said tenderly. "I have everything planned out."

Shaman went behind their small house and returned with something he had secretly built. It was a pole with two large baskets. Each basket hung by ropes from opposite ends of the pole. Carefully he lifted his mother into one basket and his father into the other basket.

The mother and father burst into tears.

"We're too heavy for you!" They sobbed. "You can't walk for miles and miles carrying us!"

"I have lots of strength," Shaman insisted. "I'll carry you as if I'm carrying flowers."

Mother and father, then, with deepest love, each placed their hands together and blessed their son and blessed the Lord for giving them such a son and asked the Lord to give him strength.

Don't think that only saints can give blessings. Anyone who loves you can give you a blessing. The blessing comes from their heart and so it comes from God. One who receives such a blessing is truly fortunate.

So on this auspicious day, Shaman put his parents on his shoulders and started on the pilgrimage.

"Most merciful, Lord," he prayed as they left the village. "Have mercy on me, that I may bring my parents back to this same spot after our pilgrimage."

Days and days passed. Months passed and Shaman walked on, carrying his parents like flowers, never complaining. He suffered at times from the heavy sun and sometimes his feet were sore and swollen or infected with thorns and it rained, but his mind never wavered, not once. Nothing could change his mind. No weakness could shake his resolve.

By the grace of the Lord, he completed the pilgrimage and they returned to their village and everyone celebrated their return. We can only imagine the divine joy that these three souls felt after such an experience.

Our parents have given us so much protection and help. Can there be a greater irreligious act than to forget our obligations to them?

STORY #27

When we're angry, we're meditating. We're holding on to one thought line in a powerful way. We're absorbed by it, engrossed in it. All other thoughts are forgotten. Similarly, when we're absorbed in sexual thoughts, we're also meditating. But the meditation of the yogi is satvic, that means 'pure.' It doesn't cause excitement or disturbance in the mind or imbalance in the body. It increases self-control. We should meditate on the higher things to obtain peace, bliss, and happiness.

BHARAT MUNI AND THE DEER

ONCE IN INDIA THERE was a great yogi named Bharat Muni. He was a muni, a yogi of a very high nature. He lived in a small hut in the forest and ate the fruit and vegetables that he gathered in the woods.

One day he came to the bank of a river. A short distance away he saw a lion chasing a deer. The deer was pregnant. She jumped into the water and swam to the opposite shore and escaped from the lion, but in the process she lost her baby.

The baby cried, but the mother ran away terrified by the lion.

Bharat Muni's heart melted. He forgot all about his morning prayers. He forgot all about his meditation time. He rushed to the side of the fawn and gently caressed the baby's head. The tiny deer looked up at Bharat Muni with beautiful, soft eyes. The eyes of a fawn are famous for their gentleness and this great yogi fell in love with the fawn.

With great tenderness, Bharat Muni picked up the fawn and brought the small deer to his hut. He fed the deer and totally took care of her and within no time he was so enchanted with the deer that he forgot about his meditation time. He spent his whole day playing with the baby and looking after it.

Soon he was talking to the deer and the deer loved it, too. She would come and sit on Bharat Muni's lap and they were both happy.

Now how can this happen? How can a great yogi like Bharat Muni who had meditated for years forget about his meditation time for a deer?

The answer is that Bharat Muni had meditated for so long that whatever he did he completely threw his mind in that direction. It didn't matter if he was eating, or gathering wood, or walking to the river, or taking care of a baby deer. Whatever he did, his mind was totally there, one pointed.

So the baby deer had become the object of his meditation now and even though he was close to mukti, which means liberation, he didn't attain liberation in that life because he had lost his focus. He was meditating on the wrong thing.

A short time later Bharat Muni left his body still saying,

"Deer, deer, come to me!"

And the Compassionate Lord allowed Bharat Muni to be born a deer in his next incarnation. This is the ending told in India. Bharat Muni went from a yogi to a deer!

STORY #28

There may be 25 pots of water on a table, but if you're not thirsty what good are the pots? Likewise, if you're not thirsty for spiritual growth, what good is the Guru who is a pot of divine knowledge? So first we must be thirsty. Then we must prepare ourselves to receive the teachings. What good is an expensive musical instrument in the hands of a child?

THE DISCIPLE WHO LIKED MICE

ONCE THERE WAS A high master who liked to teach from the scriptures. One day he was teaching his top students from the Darshan Shastra. He had one student who he loved very much, but who had no ability at all to understand this scripture. But because the master loved him, he allowed the student to sit with the other disciples.

During the lesson, the master focused intently on those disciples capable of understanding and paid little attention to the young student.

"Why is Guruji acting like this?" The young disciple said to himself. "He doesn't pay any attention to me."

A few days later, the master was in a playful mood and the young disciple thought now is a good time to talk to him about this.

"Why don't you teach me the Darshan Shastra like you do the others?" He asked. "You don't pay any attention to me."

"My son," the Guru said kindly. "You're too young. The thoughts expressed in that Shastra are beyond your capacity right now."

"No! No!" The disciple said. "Teach me like you do the others. Please."

The master thought a minute. He didn't want to discourage his disciple so he said,

"Go get your book, then."

Immediately the young disciple ran off and came back with his book. He sat down reverently in front of his Guru prepared to listen to every word.

"Open your book to the first page," the Guru said. The Guru had no book because he knew all the pages by heart.

"Now listen to what I say."

The book was written in sutras, very short, mantra-like phrases. Sometimes there were only three words in a sutra, but these three words contained everything needed to be known or understood on that topic. Everything was reduced to its essence.

The Guru started with the first sutra on page one. He was old and had taught these sutras many times and he immediately closed his eyes and became one-pointed, deep in meditation. Gradually his voice slowed down and he taught slowly. One word. Then a long pause. Another word. Then another long pause.

The disciple listened carefully for two or three minutes. But he couldn't understand at all what the Guru was talking about or why it took him so long to speak just a few words.

So he got restless and he looked here and there. At times his Guru would raise his voice and speak with great feeling, but the disciple couldn't understand any of it no matter how hard he tried.

There was a little hole in the wall. All of a sudden the disciple saw a mouse run into the hole. Then he saw another mouse poke his head out and the two mice started playing with each other, and this absorbed the disciple's mind completely. He watched in total delight as the mice played.

The Guru continued teaching and the disciple continued watching the mice.

When the lesson was over, the Guru asked,

"My son. Did you understand the lesson?"

"No, the tail is out!" The disciple replied.

"What are you talking about?" The Guru asked. "What tail?"

"Over there!" The disciple said.

The Guru looked at the wall and saw a mousetail sticking out from a hole and he burst into laughter! He knew from the beginning that such a lesson was too difficult for this disciple, but he taught him anyway, out of love. He had spoken just to please him and bring him happiness.

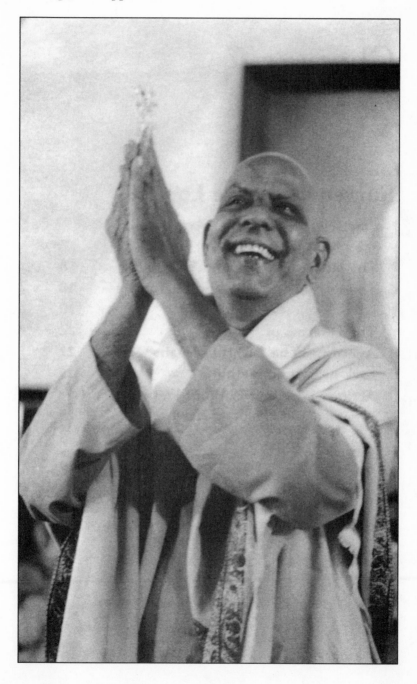

STORY #29

JESUS AND A STORY OF MERCY

(Swami Kripalu's interpretation of St. John, Chapter 8.)

Christmas, 1977

JESUS CAME DOWN FROM the mountain in the morning and came to the temple. A huge crowd had gathered to hear him because he was a great teacher.

After he spoke, everyone went home and Jesus was alone.

Before Jesus could leave, however, a group of scholars and Pharisees entered the temple with a woman who had been caught in the act of adultery. Jesus recognized that these men had come in order to test him with a complicated question.

Jesus sat quietly. The Pharisees and scholars made a circle around him. The guilty woman stood in one corner keeping her face down with shame.

The master scholar of the group addressed Jesus:

"Teacher, this woman has disobeyed the rules of religion by committing adultery. Moses has given a commandment that such a woman must be stoned to death. We have approached you to know your opinion of this."

Jesus looked from the Pharisees to the adulteress. He then looked down at his own feet. With his head bowed, he fell into deep thought.

After some moments, he spoke.

"If there is a command of religion or a rule of law, its main purpose is to benefit the individual, society, or nation. In order to protect our way of life, punishment is required of the criminal. On the other hand, there must be mercy or an understanding of the humanity in us all, in each judgment.

Each society or nation is like a family. No one can give judgment with only the words of law. It's necessary to consider the circumstances of the situation in order to make a proper judgment. In addition, there will be no similarity in different countries or in different periods of time in the judgment that one makes. It's necessary to consider these differences when making a judgment.

For these reasons, we must carefully interpret the words of the great masters. There's the possibility of doing injustice in the name of justice, by simply reading the words of the great masters."

Jesus was quiet. He looked down and went into deep thought.

The Pharisees didn't understand his words. They thought that he didn't answer their question. They knew that if Jesus went against one of the commandments of Moses, the whole society would go against him.

"What, then, is your opinion?" A Pharisee asked.

Jesus heard his words and sensed his wrong motive, yet he continued thinking quietly as the finger of his right hand wrote in the ground by his side.

Jesus continued in deep thought for about 10 minutes.

The questioners asked him repeatedly for an answer.

At last, the thought stream of Jesus Christ arrived at the feet of Truth. His finger stopped moving on the ground as he received the truth. He sat up straight, as if justice itself had risen. He gave his opinion firmly:

"Dear followers of religion, please listen. The commandment of Moses is true. It cannot be disobeyed. The adulteress has sinned. Let any of you who has not sinned get up and stone her."

Jesus again bowed his head and he again wrote with his finger on the ground beside him as before. Is he not sure of his Truth? Is he checking it again? No, he has given his opinion and is returning to meditation.

The Pharisees were speechless. They were amazed. There was nothing left for them to say. One by one they stood up and left the temple. Within a short time, the entire group had gone leaving only two people remaining.

Jesus came out of meditation. There was no one in the temple except Jesus and the adulteress.

"Are they gone?" Jesus asked the adulteress.

"Yes," she answered.

"You weren't punished by anyone?"

"No," she answered.

"Then I can't say you're guilty. Go home joyfully, but remember my words. The temple of God is an ocean of holiness. Those who bathe in it with faith become holy. If you believe, your sins are purified. Always pray to God and keep yourself away from sin. I can't judge you for your past. Whenever you repent, you're purified."

STORY #30

On this beautiful morning you have reminded me of my beloved Gurudev. I thank you for that. Beloved Gurudev is my whole life. I'm alive on this earth only by His grace. My life would be meaningless without His love. I can't describe in words to you the nature of my Gurudev, who He was, what He was about. An artist may paint a picture of the sun, but no matter how good the picture is, that sun can't give light. No matter how I describe my Gurudev to you, you can only know Him through your imagination, which will never be the true picture of Him.

HOW I MET MY GURUDEV

I WAS YOUNG, ONLY 19 years old. I was extremely ambitious, but unable to attain what I really wanted, so I was disillusioned with life. From childhood I had been attracted to the feet of the Lord. The Lord was my solace, my support, and my life. I didn't know anything about sadhana at that time, so I used to worship God according to the tradition of my family.

After the death of my father, our family was thrown into poverty. I couldn't bear this pain, even though I was only 7 years old, so I made a firm vow that I would give my whole life to God and bring happiness to my suffering family.

I had to drop out of school even though I was a bright, motivated student. I loved to read, but our family needed money and I tried to do what I could.

When I was 19, I left for Bombay to try to find work, but my heart was full of darkness. Finally, I decided it was better to commit suicide and go home to the Lord. I planned the whole thing; I was going to throw myself under a train.

Our family worshipped the Lord in the form of the Divine Mother, so I went into a nearby temple to worship the Divine Mother for the last time before I killed myself.

It was about 9:00 o'clock at night. I entered the temple in total despair and my heart melted and tears rolled down my cheeks. I went to the altar and bowed down and burst into even more tears. I had come simply to say good-by. I was going to kill myself at midnight. The statue of the Divine Mother didn't look like stone to me; She looked alive. Her eyes were full of love and I was there to ask permission for what I was about to do.

The caretaker of the temple knew me and he tried to console me, but he couldn't. I just kept crying. And at that auspicious moment, my Gurudev entered the temple. I was thirsty for knowledge. I had been to many different saints. I had read books about mantra and tantra and magic and had visited all the saints, but I had never trusted any of them. For me a guru had to be someone I could give my whole life to, nothing less, so I had given up trying to find a guru. I had totally stopped thinking about it.

Gurudev entered the temple and he said just one word, "Son."

I can't describe to you the sweetness of that word, no matter how hard I try. He lovingly placed his hand on my head and then he hugged me.

"Come with me," he said.

He was a total stranger and yet His love was so profound that I immediately yielded to Him. We walked outside the temple and then he sat down on the steps of one of the shops.

"My son," he said. "Are you going to commit suicide? Suicide isn't good."

"Oh, no!" I said. "No! No! No! I would never do that!"

I wasn't a dishonest person or a liar. I was just in shock that someone knew my deepest thoughts.

"You're a sadhak," he said. "And you must speak the truth. Tonight you were going to throw yourself under a train." And then he described my whole scheme.

When he was finished, I bowed down to him and touched his feet.

"Please forgive this child," I said.

"Come and see me next Thursday," he said, and he gave me an address.

Thursday is the day of the guru in India and I discovered that he always gave darshan on that day. But I arrived late. I tried hard to be on time, but I failed to do so. I bought a garland of flowers for five rupees with great love. I had little money and you could buy a nice garland for one rupee, but I selected a beautiful garland for five rupees with great love.

I placed the garland around his neck and then gave him a dandwood pranam, lying down completely flat on my stomach. He looked at me and the nectar of love flowed from his pure, beautiful eyes.

"My son, swami, you have come," he said, stroking my head.

The word, swami, surprised me.

"I'm not a swami," I said.

"My son, I've called you swami because you're going to be a swami in the future."

"Me?" I gasped. "Oh, no! I don't think so! I can't do all that begging!"

"It's true that swamis beg for food," he said. "But they aren't beggars as you understand it. They're beggars of love. You're going to give your love to the world and you're going to receive love from the world."

I was crying now and even though I was crying, I was happy.

Gurudev had known that I would be late that day and he had instructed the gatekeeper to keep the gate open for me, even though he normally ended darshan promptly.

"One child will come," he had told them, "and he will be late, but let him in."

Then he had saved a spot next to him for me to sit, while all the other disciples had to sit at a distance. But there was great joy on their faces.

"I've come here for one young disciple who will come to us today," he had told them. "I'll initiate him into swamihood and then I'll leave. He'll become a great yogi."

Gurudev attracted me to his feet when I was 19. I stayed with him for a year and a quarter. It's by his grace that I've been able to maintain this sadhana for so many years. There's only one thing that I want to do with my life, and that's to do sadhana for as far as it will take me. I have no attraction left for money, fame, or name. My only desire is to remember the name of God.

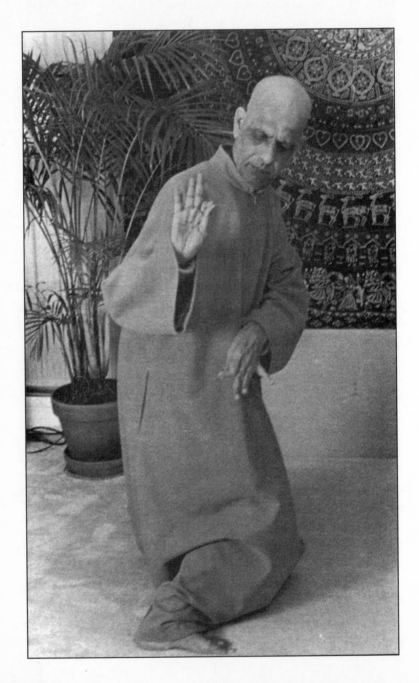

STORY #31

Today you have all gathered to celebrate my birthday. It's the start of my 67th year, and I bless you with all my heart. I'm an old sadhak wanting only final liberation. You call me Dada, or Grandfather, and it isn't proper for me to cry in front of you, but every word I speak, every gaze from my eyes, is full of love for you. I don't speak English, but can any language truly express love? No, love is expressed only through the heart and the eyes.

Life is the flow of our own existence between birth and death. Some people say that life is an endless circle of mistakes which can never be prevented, or that life is a chaotic mixture of happiness and unhappiness. Other people take a different view. They say that life means love; life means progress; life means light; life means evolution.

Both groups agree, however, that life means struggle, that we all must struggle. This world is a battlefield. Anyone born has to be a warrior, whether you are boy or girl, man or woman, young or old, king or beggar, literate or illiterate, saint or sinner, our major dharma or duty in this world is to fight. The compassionate Lord has one special Angel to help with our fight. This is the Angel of Struggle.

THE STORY OF SWAMI VIVEKANANDA

ONCE IN INDIA THERE was a boy named Narendra Kumar. From birth he had a good character. His early life was happy. He received a good education and had an intellectual mind.

But then the family situation changed. The family became poor. More and more his mother, who now lived in poverty, looked to Narendra to help their family. He was a bright, well-educated, extremely capable young man, and she was certain, through God's grace, that he would receive a nice job soon and save their family. Then he would marry and her daughter-in-law would come to live with her, and she would have a beautiful grandchild. And then, as she neared death, she would say to her son:

"Narendra, because of you, my unhappy heart has received peace. I give my blessings to you and your family with my whole heart. My last desire is to live in the holy place of Kashi and leave my body there."

That was her plan.

But Almighty God had a different plan for young Narendra, one that wasn't quite so ordinary, one that would bestow great happiness on many, many people.

So one day God called Struggle to His side.

"Struggle! My dear, Angel!" He said, "Come here!" and He whispered secret commands into her ear.

"Now, go!" He said, "And visit young Narendra!"

By this time, Narendra Kumar had finished his studies in the university. While he was a university student, he had mostly studied complicated scriptures, like the Upanishads and other philosophies. He had also come into contact with numerous saints, and was more attracted to the spiritual world than the material world.

He completed his studies and began to search for a job. At first he was certain he would find a good job quickly. But this didn't happen and he became frustrated. Finally, he became ashamed of himself and lost all self-confidence. Here he was with a high education, yet no one would hire him. What was wrong with him, he asked? He had no income at all, nothing, and his family had no savings.

Then he discovered one day that his mother had stopped eating so she could feed him the little food they had left in the house. This was intolerable. So every morning, with greater determination, he renewed his job search.

His family lived in Calcutta, so there was no lack of public transportation or restaurants, but he had no money for food or transportation. So each day he walked and drank water.

Who would like such an unhappy life?

Each evening he returned home. But before he entered his house, he rested his sore feet, wiped the look of dejection and failure off his face, and walked through the door only when he felt strong again. Then in a sweet voice, full of love, he told his mother the same lie.

"Mother, I'm sorry I'm late tonight. I met an old friend and he invited me to his house for supper, so don't worry about me, my stomach is full. Everything will be fine, don't worry. I had several good interviews today. We must be patient a little while longer. Please eat now. I'm going to my room to read for awhile."

These were such unhappy days for Narendra Kumar. The Angel of Struggle had firmly shut all the doors to material prosperity. God, Himself, had ordered this. The only door left open to young Narendra was the door to the spiritual path.

One day Narendra reached the Holy feet of Shri Ramakrishna Paramahansa. Narendra had known about Ramakrishna's popularity for a long time, but had never met him. He experienced peace from the darshan of Shri Ramakrishna, and he asked Ramakrishna the same question that he had asked numerous other saints:

"Have you seen God?"

Ramakrishna's face lit with a sweet smile and the nectar of compassion flowed from his eyes. With pure love, he answered Narendra's question with a question,

"Do you desire to see God?"

"Yes, please," Narendra replied.

"This is the best thing," Ramakrishna said.

That day, Narendra received perfect comfort from his conversation with Ramakrishna. He went back to him and grew in spiritual knowledge and detachment from the world. One day he took sanyas initiation, total renunciation with perfect brahmacharya, and Shri Ramakrishna gave him the name Swami Vivekananda.

Today millions of people know of Swami Vivekananda. Anyone can read his biography and discourses and become acquainted with his unique personality. This is the same brilliant swami who felt useless as a young man, unable to get a job, walking alone on the streets of Calcutta penniless and poor, lying to his mother so she could eat instead of him. Did he not have greatness in him then? If Struggle had not closed the door to material success, but had given him a nice job instead, perhaps his life would have been different.

Swami Vivekananda was inspired to come to the America.

"Swamiji," everyone said who met him, "Please speak in Chicago at the Parliament of World Religions." At that time, no one knew him. He was given only 15 minutes to speak, but he rose from his seat and spoke so sweetly about God that all the listeners were spellbound by his words. After that, his popularity spread all over America.

Just as our food won't digest properly without exercise, so too our life won't develop properly without struggle. The outward form of struggle may appear cruel, but its inner nature is not malicious. She enters our life without invitation and does whatever she pleases, but she blesses us with true knowledge, the knowledge we each need at that time in our life. How skillful she is! What a beautiful sculptor!

STORY #32

*Once a man entered a town and asked a small child: "Have any
great men and women ever been born in your town?" "Oh, no!"
The child answered, "Only babies are born in our town." And
so it is with faith and devotion. The love between a guru and a
disciple doesn't happen all of a sudden. It starts small, like a baby,
and grows bigger and bigger and it develops best when we have a
chance to live with the guru and observe his or her pure character.
When this faith and devotion matures, it's a great blessing, because
it helps us progress on the spiritual path during difficult times.*

THE DISCIPLE AND THE COBRA

ONCE THERE WAS A saint in India who led a simple life
in the forest. He had one disciple. After living together
for many years, the disciple had complete faith in his
guru. To him, his guru was mother, father, brother, sister, friend,
everything.

One evening, the guru was teaching his disciple. When it got
dark, the guru said,

"My, son. Go to bed now. I'll stay up a little longer."

The disciple fell asleep under a nearby tree. The guru finished
his evening meditation and when he opened his eyes he saw a huge
cobra slowly moving toward his sleeping disciple. The guru was
certain that if a cobra this big bit his disciple that his disciple would
die.

The guru folded his hands in prayer and approached the
snake.

"Nagdev," he said. Here nag means cobra, and dev means divine, so he addressed the cobra this way, very respectfully. "Where
are you going?"

"I'm going to drink the blood of your disciple," the cobra said.

"That's all you want?" The guru asked, "Just his blood?"

"Yes, just his blood," the cobra said.

"And if I give you his blood, will you be satisfied?"

"Yes," the cobra said. "That will satisfy my revenge from a past lifetime."

"Then wait a minute," the guru said. "Don't bite him." The guru took a small bowl and a knife and walked over to the tree. The disciple was sleeping on his back, and the guru sat on his chest with the knife.

But at that moment the disciple woke up. In the moonlight he saw someone sitting on his chest with a knife in his hand, and he was afraid. But then he realized that it was his guru, so he simply closed his eyes again.

"From what part of his body do you want the blood?" The guru asked.

"From his throat," the cobra replied.

The guru made a small cut in his disciple's throat and caught the blood in the bowl. The disciple made no sound. He just accepted the pain with eyes still closed. The guru brought the blood to the cobra and the snake drank it and left.

The next morning the disciple showed no curiosity at all about what had happened. He asked nothing about the incident. Five or six months passed and still the disciple never questioned his guru.

"My son," the guru said one day. "That night when I cut your throat, don't you want to know why?"

"No," the disciple said. "It doesn't matter to me. You're my guru. You're everything to me. So when you were cutting my throat, I knew you were doing something good for me."

Faith and devotion that can't be disturbed or destroyed even under trying conditions is true faith. This is shraddha in the scriptures. It means powerful faith that can't be extinguished. This is the flame that we should keep burning in our hearts.

STORY #33

When someone we love dies, the pain of separation is difficult to bear. Slowly after many months, as we gradually involve our mind with new activities, our suffering lightens. The only necessity is a change of thought. If we could bring about this change within a few days, we would only suffer a few days. We could say, if we don't want to see the scenes in the west, all we have to do is turn our face to the east. How simple it appears, yet how difficult this is to accomplish.

THE SAINT WHO COULDN'T PRACTICE WHAT HE PREACHED

ONCE THERE WAS A rich man in India with only one son. The rich man grew old and one day his son died. The old man cried so heavily that he couldn't stop. Relatives and friends came to his side and tried to console him, but nothing worked. He just kept crying and crying. Soon his friends started thinking that if we can't get him to stop crying, he'll die soon, too.

There was a great learned man living in the town, a saint, well respected by everyone. His words and presence were powerful so several relatives of the old man went to the saint and asked for his help.

"Please help us," they said. "Our dear relative is so distraught over the death of his son that he won't stop crying. Perhaps you could explain to him the nature of death and help him overcome his loss."

"Yes, I can do that," the saint said. He was very confident. "I'll visit him and everything will be alright."

When the saint approached the house of the rich man, he could hear the old man crying loudly inside. The saint knocked on the door. The rich man knew about the visit and opened the door, quieting down for a moment. He gave the saint a seat and then burst into tears again, wailing loudly in front of the saint.

"This death has occurred by the will of God," the saint said sweetly. "You must accept it. The soul of your son is eternal, undying. He lives still in soul form. This body is like a garment of clothes. Just as we change clothes, so we change our form at death, that's all. Your son is still alive and you will see him again."

The saint kept talking like this, very sweetly, explaining all the beautiful things from the Shastras and other scriptures. The businessman finally quieted down and stopped crying.

Two years went by. The businessman got over the death of his son and became busy with other activities in his old age. Then one day he happened to pass by the house of the saint again. There was a large crowd of people outside the door.

"What's going on here?" The old man asked. "What's wrong? Why are you all standing here looking so worried?"

Before anyone could answer, however, the old man heard someone crying loudly inside. He recognized the voice of the saint and realized the saint was crying uncontrollably about something. He was stunned. How could someone as learned and wise as this saint be crying so loudly over anything?

So he went inside and found the saint wailing loudly in deep pain and sorrow.

"Dear sir?" He asked softly. "Why are you crying like this?"

"I've been suffering from tuberculosis now for two years," the saint replied. "A kind doctor advised me to drink goat's milk to help my condition, so I bought a goat and drank her milk each day. It was such a wonderful goat and today she died."

"You're crying over a dead goat!" The old man asked incredulously.

"Old man," the saint said. "The wife who died was yours, but the goat was mine!"

STORY #34

Sanatana Dharma, the eternal religion of India, allows devotees to worship whatever form or aspect of God that is most meaningful to them. So India is full of statues. Isn't this idol worship? How can there be life in stone? Have you ever watched a child play with a doll? She treats the doll as if the doll were alive. She talks to the doll and feeds and dresses the doll and comforts the doll when the doll cries. For her the doll is alive. In a similar manner, for the people of India, their chosen form of God is alive, too, and they worship that form daily in a ceremony called, puja.

A WOMAN REMEMBERS HER SON

ONCE A YOUNG WOMAN came crying to me.

"My son has died," she sobbed. "He was only five years old."

I could do nothing except let her cry. She was in great pain. It was her only child.

When she returned home, she gathered all of her son's things and put them in a chest, all of his clothes and toys.

One year went by. Two years went by. Three years went by.

Then one day she was looking for something and she accidentally opened the chest. There in front of her were the tiny shoes of her son, his tiny socks, his tiny shirts, his tiny cap, and all the toys she had given him. She picked up the toys and remembered each one, when she had given the toy and for what occasion. And she looked at the pictures again, when her son was born and each year of his short life, and she saw him smiling in the pictures and saw him in her arms again, and she was overwhelmed and began crying and held the pictures to her chest as if she was holding him again. Her son came to life in her heart when she saw all of these things.

Many people in India have this much devotion for God. Their chosen form of God isn't just a statue of stone; the statue opens their heart and their devotion becomes a form of meditation and it purifies their mind.

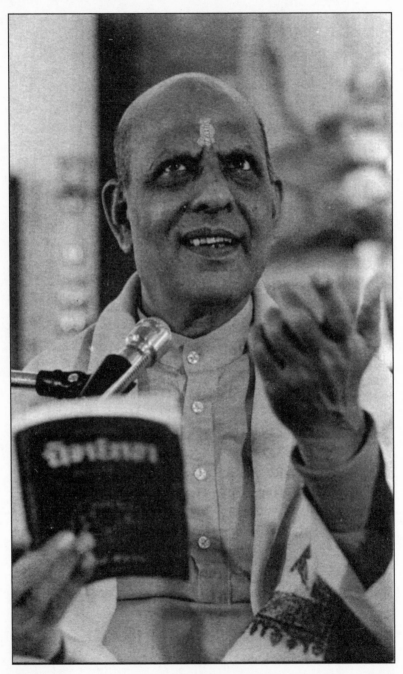

STORY #35

Imagine if a train decided that it didn't need the tracks? That it would just go wherever it wanted to? There would be an accident, of course. Likewise if we give up the tracks of religion, we'll have an accident, too. Don't let these accidents happen to you. Stay awake and let your life be guided by the tracks of religion, even though it may be hard at times.

THE STRONG WRESTLER

ONCE THERE WAS A strong wrestler. He was huge, a massive athlete, and very strong. He could lift a hundred pounds with one hand and throw it wherever he wanted to.

One day someone said something to him that he didn't like and he got angry, quickly, just like that, and he exploded with rage.

"Do you know who you're talking to?" He hollered at the person. "Do you know how strong I am? I can pick up a heavy stone and throw it anywhere I want to and I can do that to you, too, you tiny little thing! So watch your mouth!"

A saint was standing nearby and heard all of this. He approached the strong wrestler and spoke to him with great love.

"Can you really pick up a large stone and throw it anywhere you want to?" He asked gently.

"Yes! Anywhere!" The wrestler replied, still angry.

"Can't you also, then, take this little bit of abuse and throw it away? Your body is strong, but your mind is weak. Can't it carry even this much weight?"

Religion is like a needle; it brings two pieces, two people, together. Non-religion is like a scissors; it divides and makes two out of one.

STORY #36

THE DEATH OF LORD BUDDHA

ONE MORNING, ANAND, THE disciple of Lord Buddha was meditating. As his meditation was ending, he had a vision of the sun setting. Normally this wouldn't be upsetting since the sun sets everyday, but today this vision shook his body. He trembled all over and tears poured from his eyes.

The meditation continued and Anand saw the light from a lamp go out. Furthermore, the ghee in the jar was gone and the lamp couldn't be relit. Then the entire scene became pitch black and there was darkness everywhere.

Anand was a high disciple of Lord Buddha and thus he was an unattached monk. Restraint was his temperament. Lord Buddha, himself, had given him his name, Anand, which means Bliss. After meditating for years under the direction of such a high master, few things could disturb his peaceful mind.

What caused this disturbance, then? Where did it come from? Was it a premonition? He decided to discuss the matter with Lord Buddha, himself.

But today was Anand's day to visit the city and he had little time, so he quickly approached Lord Buddha for morning darshan and decided to wait until he returned to discuss the disturbance in his meditation.

Lord Buddha blessed him and Anand got up to leave, but his feet froze and his entire body shook again and his heart screamed a silent scream of intolerable pain. Clouds of tears poured from the sky of his eyes. He had never kept any secret from his Guru, yet he still wished to maintain silence about his meditation until he had returned from the city.

Anand walked toward the door, but then his heart begged him to turn once more and look upon the face of his Guru. He turned and the compassionate eyes of Lord Buddha fell on him again and overwhelmed him with love.

Then with sad steps, Anand left for the city.

Noontime came and Lord Buddha left to collect alms. A poor person offered him alms that day which contained dried poisonous mushrooms by mistake. After finishing his lunch, the Lord returned to his residence. Within an hour or two, the poison had spread throughout his entire body. The pain became intense, yet the Lord's face remained tranquil. He was a stoic; therefore he silently welcomed the pain.

It was obvious now to his disciples that Lord Buddha had been poisoned. The news spread throughout the city and thousands of feet ran toward the dying Lord. Thousands of eyes filled with tears and thousands of hearts grieved.

Lord Buddha, however, was omnipotent so surely he must have desired to withdraw himself from God's divine play, otherwise such an accident with mushrooms could never have happened.

The poor man who had offered the Buddha the mushrooms also heard the news. He ran and collapsed at the lotus feet of Lord Buddha and repeatedly begged forgiveness. The Lord comforted him with total affection.

Anand, too, heard the news while he was still in the city and he rushed back to the monastery. Lord Buddha lay dying in seclusion. Other disciples were guarding the door to his room to keep the grieving people away, as everything was in chaos.

Anand was a close disciple, so he entered the room to serve his master. He bowed with great reverence and now he understood the significance of the setting sun in his meditation and the extinguished flame.

With great tenderness he sat in front of his dying Lord and he tried not to cry, but he didn't succeed in the least. Great sobs of despair burst from his heart, as if he was crying for all the grieving masses outside the monastery.

Lord Buddha allowed him to cry with great patience.

When Anand finally had no more tears, their eyes met. Anand saw that Lord Buddha's face was radiant and in that moment, a huge ocean of love poured from the Lord's eyes, as if the entire heart of the Buddha had migrated into his eyes.

"Anand," Lord Buddha whispered with such sweetness that the memory of that word and the way it was spoken would forever be with Anand.

"Bhagwan," Anand whispered back, still grieving, "What happened? Part of me says that this was just an accident, that no one would poison you intentionally. Yet, I'm not convinced."

"The deed wasn't intentional," the Buddha said. "And it isn't my task to ponder his part. I'm only evaluating my part. I firmly believe that this incident is the result of my karma. Only after I have suffered through it will I be free of it. So hold no hatred towards him. If you hold hatred, new karma will be created in a vicious circle and it will be an obstacle on the path to your own liberation."

Equanimity is the foundation of greatness and those who are able to behave favorably in even unfavorable situations are indeed great men.

Anand, however, was still a disciple, not a master, so he had doubts.

"My Lord," he said. "I understand the truth in your words, yet my heart is still angry. This is such a vicious incident. Isn't anger and bitterness a natural reaction?"

Fierce flames from the poison burned in every atom of the Buddha's body, but the Lord was in deep contemplation. He was a great stoic and his mind and body were strong and capable of tolerating any type of pain. Great masters don't allow their minds to go unrestrained toward either pleasure or pain. This is equanimity.

"Son," Lord Buddha said. "It's normal to hold hateful feelings when these things happen. To suppress such feelings is also wrong. Eventually learn to tolerate the situation, believing it be the result of one's previous karma."

Anand bowed down at his master's holy feet with faith and devotion. Years ago he had offered his life to the Buddha and today he offered his life again, but this time with greater understanding. Now he never even considered saying, Please bless me, anymore.

He had complete faith now that the Lord's strong grace would always be with him, a treasure house of blessings.

Anand left the room to allow Lord Buddha silence, but he felt as he walked out that Lord Buddha was walking with him.

A few minutes later, Lord Buddha left his body and entered Nirvana.

Three days later, Anand awoke suddenly from a deep sleep. He looked around and remembered where he had laid down to rest, next to a riverbank. In the distance he could see a chain of mountains studded with a canopy of green trees. Rivers flowed easily from the mountains in divine beauty.

It was dusk and the sun glowed with a deep red hue as it gradually descended from the blue sky. Was it truly the sun? No, Anand thought, it's my Lord, himself, gradually withdrawing his radiance from this earth.

Tears filled his eyes and he slipped into meditation.

"Anand?" He heard a voice say sweetly.

"Yes," he replied quickly, as every atom in his body recognized the voice and surged with a reply.

"Do you believe me to be dead?"

"Bhagwan, permanent separation from the body is called death, is it not?"

"Anand, you haven't yet become truly Anand, true Bliss. Only a genuine monk can be considered Anand. You have remained worldly, as yet, and that's the reason you're lamenting. Give up your despair."

"I hate the word death!" Anand shouted. "That's the reason for my despair!"

"Dear monk, you haven't yet realized the final truth. Listen! As long as my yogic principles live and as long as my system of sadhana lives, I will also live. Death of the truth is my death. Since truth is eternal, I'm also eternal. I, the Buddha, was merely a seed. At the end of my sadhana, a huge Buddha tree has sprouted from this seed. On its countless small and large branches and subbranches innumerable Buddha seeds have budded. Anand, in the future huge forests of Buddhas will flourish. I believe this occurrence to be the cause of my immortality. This is not ego. One in who ego resides can never be called a yogi."

Anand almost drowned in the river of Lord Buddha's teachings.

"Bhagwan," he whispered. "My aching heart has received complete consolation. My Lord, now I will be able to walk upon the path lit by you for countless years to come. With your grace, I'll reach the final destination."

STORY #37

Many years ago when I was sitting in meditation, I chanted this same Ram dhun that I chanted for you this morning. The tune emerged automatically from within. I didn't try to chant it or arrange the words or the tune. It just came spontaneously from within. This is called anahat nad, or spontaneous sound. This happens in yoga sadhana when the prana and apana both begin to rise up. When they join together and work in the visuddha chakra, or throat chakra, sound is produced. The yogi spontaneously chants Om, Ram, and the immortal mantras such as the Gayatri and Om Namo Bhagavate Vasudevaya, your mantra. These are divine sounds to the yogi and so the yogi says these sounds are from God. When we use sound willfully to create music we can enchant our mind and make it one pointed. It's useful then as a tool for meditation. We can even use sound as a friend in a difficult situation, which reminds me of a funny story.

THE WOMAN AND THE TRUCK DRIVER

ONCE A YOUNG SISTER was driving on a narrow mountain road. The road was so narrow that there was only one lane. She was all alone. It was night time, very dark, and her car broke down.

"Now what will I do?" She said. "There's no one around to help me."

She tried fixing her car, but couldn't. So she got back in her car to rest until help came.

It was late and she was tired so she fell asleep.

Eventually a truck arrived. The driver saw the car blocking his way and someone sleeping and he became angry. There was no way he could get around the car because the road was too narrow, so he honked his horn. Then in anger he kept honking it again and again.

The sister woke up and now she was scared. She was all alone on a mountain road and in a bad situation A strange man was angry at her, honking his horn and wanting her to move, yet she couldn't move her car.

Getting up her courage, the young sister opened her car door and approached the truck driver.

"Dear brother," she said with a smiling face. "Would you please help me? I'm having car trouble. I've tried, but I don't know what's wrong with my car. I'm sorry I'm in your way."

Listening to her kind words and seeing her desperate situation, the truck driver climbed down and agreed to help.

"Thank you," she said, climbing into his truck. "You keep trying to repair my car and I'll keep honking."

They both laughed and all the tension in the situation ended. The kind truck driver fixed her car and they both continued on their way.

STORY #38

Pray to the Lord daily and accept happiness and unhappiness as the grace of the Lord. The Lord keeps the sun in the sky so everyone can have heat and light and keeps the moon in the sky so everyone can have coolness at night. The Lord opens the flowers and allows them to bloom and then closes and dries them up. All of these things happen by the will of the Lord and we are His children and He loves us. He doesn't want us to suffer or to be anxious. So rest, rest at His holy feet knowing you are cared for.

MY FIRST MEAL AS A SWAMI

THE SAINT WHO GAVE me swami initiation was Shantanandiji Maharaj. I was 32 years old at the time. With this initiation, I vowed to be detached from everything: my relatives, my home, my town, everything.

I left the ashram the next day and set out on my own. I now had to beg for food and be prepared to sleep under a tree wherever my feet stopped for the day. I had never asked for alms before and I was hesitant.

"How can I beg for food?" I asked myself. I felt helpless.

I walked three or four miles and came to a small town. There was a temple there and I went in, bowed to the altar, and sat in the corner of the temple. It was exactly twelve o'clock noon and time for a meal.

I wasn't particularly hungry and was thinking to myself,

"Maybe I'll go for two or three days before I ask for food. I can make it that long. But I'll certainly have to ask for alms after four or five days."

The women of India, the mothers and sisters, are so kind that as soon as a swami asks for alms they immediately give food, no matter how poor they are, so I wasn't too concerned about food.

As I sat in the corner of the temple, I noticed there was another temple behind it. Both temples were in the same compound close to each other and a mother and her son appeared to be living in the other temple. I could see that they did the pujas in both temples.

"Mother," I heard the boy say, "Yesterday, aunty promised that she would join us for our noon meal. But she's not coming now. She says that she's already eaten. What are we going to do with this extra food?"

"Oh," the mother said. "Don't worry about it. Go and finish your puja in the other temple."

The boy walked into the temple where I was sitting and he finished the puja with great devotion. Then he saw me and hurried back to his mother.

"Mother," he said. "There's a swami sitting in the other temple."

"My son," the mother said. "This extra food that we prepared today is for him. Go and tell him not to seek alms anywhere else, because his food is already prepared."

The son quickly came to me. He bowed down.

"Please come to our home for your noon meal," he said sweetly.

There are two types of alms for swamis in India. In the first one, the swami sits and eats with the family who offered the food. In the second, the swami graciously accepts the food and then retires to a quiet place to eat alone. Both of these manners are widely accepted and understood. It's up to the saint how he or she wants to accept the alms.

I followed the boy into the other temple. The mother was standing on the temple steps with a bucket of water and she washed my feet. Then her son wiped my feet with a clean cloth and they took me inside. The mother asked me to sit on a wooden platform while she waited on me. She lit incense and doted on me like I was her own son, with so much love and devotion and I was greatly moved.

Then the mother served me sweets and they both fanned me while I ate. This was my first meal as a swami and I felt that God was already taking care of me. Tears rolled down my face when I left and I knew, then, that I would never, ever, worry about myself. The Lord is always the well-wisher of everyone and it's His goal to bring happiness to everyone.

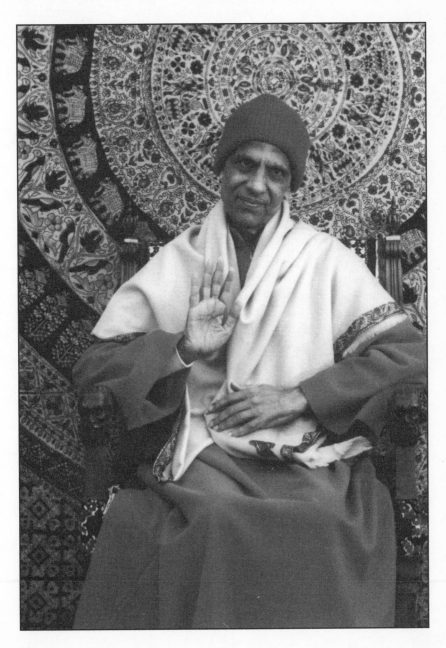

STORY #39

THE MAN WHO WAS GOING TO AMERICA

ONCE THERE WAS A well-known saint in India named Swami Ram Tirtha. He lived during the time of Swami Vivikananda. He was truly a non-attached mahatma. He decided to visit America, but before he left India, a man came up to him and asked,

"Are you really going to America?"

"Yes," he said.

"Please write to me and tell me when you're returning, as I would like to see you then."

"That's fine," Swami Ram Tirtha said.

Swami Ram Tirtha left for America, just as he had planned, and stayed a long time and created many devotees. When he returned to India, the same man found him.

"You're back from America now?" The man asked.

"Yes," Swami Ram Tirtha said.

"I'm also thinking of going to the America," the man said. "How expensive is it?"

"There's no expense at all," Swami Ram Tirtha said.

"But I'm not a swami like you," the man said. "No one will give me food, money, and passage. How can I go to America without money?"

"Brother," Swami Ram Tirtha said. "You're just thinking about going to America, so there's no expense involved. The expense comes only when you go there."

It's the same on the spiritual path. As long as we only think about going to God, there's no expense involved. The expense comes only when we decide to make the journey.

STORY #40

Whether we are born man or woman, we must be warriors if we are to arrive at the feet of the Lord. We must be patient and tireless in our effort, even when we're deceived. Mistakes committed in ignorance can hurt our progress, but they can help us, too. They teach us to recognize true knowledge and true teachers. Knowledge received through life's difficulties is precious. It's special. This knowledge is more valuable that the knowledge we receive in satsanga, which is only words and often just stored in our memory. So continue on, don't become discouraged when you're deceived. There's a funny story in India that I'll tell you about deception. I'll tell it to you as your grandfather, not as a dharma acharya, since the great masters used humor carefully because spiritual knowledge was sacred.

THE ACHARYA WITHOUT A NOSE

ONCE A GREAT MASTER came to a town in India. His speaking manner was so attractive that everyone was enchanted with him.

"Beloved lovers of God," he said, "The Lord isn't far from you. He loves you and is very close to you."

A man named Augar Bhagat was in the crowd and he heard this. He was extremely dull, but he liked music and so he was in one of the chanting groups. He discovered, however, that when he sang bhajans nobody paid any attention to him. So he learned to cry. These were fake tears, but he discovered that when he sang and cried everyone thought he was crying because he missed the Lord so much, tears of separation, so they respected him and listened to his singing.

But he was simply a great actor. He learned to relax all the muscles on his face so thoroughly that it looked like he was totally sick of the world and wanted only the Lord. Then, using his will power he would open his tear glands and cry at the right time.

Augar Bhagat heard the saint say again, "The Lord isn't far from you. He loves you and is very close to you," and he said to himself,

"Augar Bhagat, you must be blind! The Lord is so close to you and yet you can't see Him?"

The saint continued with his discourse.

"The reason why you can't see the Lord even though He's so close is because of your nose. Your nose is useless. It's in the way. Unless you cut off your nose, you'll never see the Lord."

Augar Bhagat liked this explanation and smiled to himself.

"Because of this useless nose I can't see the Lord? It's that simple? Well, I can live without a nose, but I can't live without seeing the Lord. So tomorrow I'll definitely cut off my nose. It's coming between me and the Lord."

The saint continued with his discourse.

"The nose that I'm talking about isn't the nose that takes the breath in and out. The nose I'm talking about is ego. Only the devotee who cuts off the nose of ego can see the Lord."

Augar Bhagat, however, was too dull to understand this. And besides he was too busy congratulating himself. He was totally convinced that he had digested the essence of the lecture and so he happily went home.

The next morning he got up early and entered his meditation room. He bowed to the Lord, lit a ghee lamp, and finished his puja. Then he took a sharp knife and with great faith cut off his nose. He placed his nose on his altar as an offering to the Lord.

"Now!" he said, bandaging his face, "The Lord will appear to me!"

Five minutes passed, but the Lord didn't appear. Augar Bhagat changed the dressing on his face and waited again.

Hours passed. The day passed. Night passed. Three days passed. And yet he didn't see the Lord.

"The shastras, the scriptures, the saints are all liars!" He finally said, unable to wait any longer. "Even God is a lie! How will I ever be able to live in society again without a nose? Everyone will laugh at me and call me a fool!"

Soon his neighbors knocked on his door. They hadn't seen him for three days and they were worried.

"Augar Bhagat!" They called. "Are you alright?"

When no one answered they entered his home. By now Augar Bhagat had a plan. He went into his meditation room and stayed there, and when his neighbors entered the room, they found him dancing and singing in a funny nasal voice, acting as if he saw no one. He appeared to be in deep meditation unaware of his surroundings and he was chanting all the names of God. The people saw his nose on the altar and the bandage on his face and now they understood what had happened.

A close friend stopped Augar Bhagat from dancing. Augar Bhagat pretended to be coming out of deep meditation. He showed great surprise that people were in his room. He started crying and bowed down over and over to his altar, as if he was crazy with God intoxication.

"Brothers and Sisters!" he said. "How can I describe it to you! I've found the Lord and my life is finished! He's right in front of me! Oh, what a beautiful face! If you could only see it! My life is totally fulfilled!"

The people in the room scrambled to bow to him and to acknowledge him as a great devotee of the Lord now. Seeing this, Augar Bhagat said slyly to himself,

"I don't mind losing my nose now. It will make me famous."

Soon the whole town came for his darshan. Then people from other towns came to see him.

"Augar Bhagat has found the Lord!" Everyone said. "He has seen the Lord personally!"

Then people started talking about his miracles and yogic powers.

"He has created food with mantra power and fed thousands!" They said. "And he has given away bags and bags of money to the poor and piles of clothing!"

Within a few weeks people from all over brought him presents as if he were God. They brought him silk clothing, silver sandals, velvet cushions, eating utensils made of gold and silver, and rich people came to fan him. There was no end to his prosperity.

Then they asked him to give spiritual discourses.

"Beloved lovers of God," he said, "God isn't far from you. He's very close to you. Your nose is keeping you from seeing the Lord. Cut off your nose and you'll see the Lord instantly. That's how I found the Lord. I'll show anyone how to do it, but first you must take mantra diksha from me and then follow my exact instructions."

Hundreds of devotees came forth eager to see God. They bowed to Augar Bhagat, gave him gifts, received mantra diksha, and then cut off their noses.

"Fools!" Augar Bhagat told them in private. "There's no God. God doesn't exist anywhere on this earth. You can cut off your nose and your head, too, and you'll never see God. That's the spiritual truth that I have to give you. And now what are you going to do? People are going to laugh at you for the rest of your life! Now you must truly listen to me. Go out into the community and tell people that you've seen the Lord, that there's no end to your bliss, that your life is now complete, and it's all because you've cut off your nose!"

And that's what the people did. They were so angry and embarrassed that they left and went out and danced in the streets for joy and told everyone that the compassionate Lord had blessed them with His darshan and it was all because they had cut off their nose.

Within six months, Augar Bhagat had a huge following. His disciples with their cut noses said that Augar Bhagat was an incarnation of God, that he had taken away all their pain. Then they read a few yogic scriptures and they explained to everyone the science behind the teachings of Augar Bhagat.

"The yogic scriptures say that prana should enter the shushumna nadi," they explained. "The left nostril is called the ida. The right is called the pingala. When the flow of both of these nadis meets together, the third flow begins. That flow is called the shushumna nadi. That nadi is in the center, right here. By cutting off your nose, the shushumna opens up and that's the home of the Lord."

One day a great King heard about Augar Bhagat and invited him to his palace. He gave Augar Bhagat a special residence in the palace and came to him for darshan every day.

"I've offered my entire life to God," Augar Bhagat told the King. "See all the people without noses? They, too, have seen the Lord after following my instructions."

The King was ready to take mantra diksha and cut off his nose. But he had one wise minister who's job it was to protect the King from fraud.

"Beloved saint," the minister said coyly to Augar Bhagat. "Pardon me, but I don't see anything in your teachings. You can't see God by cutting off your nose. The only reason you're saying that is to save yourself the embarrassment of going through life without a nose. Otherwise people would laugh at you and say, 'Look at that fool! He cut off his nose to see God!'"

"I explained yesterday the science behind my teachings," Augar Bhagat replied. "The ancient rishis said that the Lord resides in the shushumna itself and that it's extremely difficult to pierce the ajna chakra which you must do to see the Lord. We can't pierce the ajna chakra because our nose is in the way. Ida and pingala will open when we cut off our nose. Prana will flow into shushuma and pierce the ajna chakra. Then the Lord will have to appear. He can't remain hidden any longer."

The minister had read the yogic scriptures, too, and he knew there was truth in these words. Yet, he told the King,

"Beware! Remain patient! Give this man a residence in the palace where I can watch him in secret. He's giving mantra diksha every day to dozens of people. I'll watch him and see if his initiation is true."

"Your advice is good," the King said. "And I'll come with you. Together we'll determine the character of this man."

The next day the King and his minister hid in the room where Augar Bhagat was giving mantra diksha. They saw the ceremony and watched as innocent people cut off their noses and then heard Augar Bhagat laugh at them and order them to leave the room and lie, lest people laugh at them for the rest of their lives."

The King immediately ordered Augar Bhagat arrested and put to death with no mercy, and thus the noseless path to God came to an end.

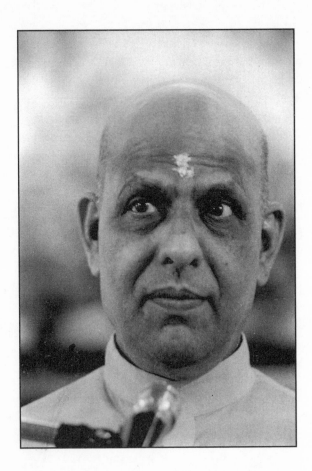

STORY #41

Wherever a lamp goes, it sheds its light. Wherever a flower goes, it sheds its fragrance. So also devotees of the Lord spread their love wherever they go.

SWAMI RAMATHIRTHA COMES TO AMERICA

YOU HAVE ALL HEARD of Swami Vivekananda. There was another saint living at the same time in India. His name was Swami Ramathirtha. One day Swami Vivekananda was visiting the state of Punjab. Swami Ramathirtha was not a swami yet; he was a professor of mathematics and a perfect follower of Vedanta. He was putting great effort into seeing God everywhere, because that is the Vedanta philosophy.

That night he heard Swami Vivekananda give a talk and he was pleased and he spoke briefly with Swami Vivekananda afterwards. Swami Ramathirtha was still in householder clothes, but Swami Vivekananda recognized his saintly nature and knew he would be a swami in the future.

After the conversation, Swami Vivekananda turned to leave. Swami Ramathirtha wanted to give him something, so he took off his beautiful gold watch and placed it in Swami Vivekananda's hand.

Swami Vivekananda looked at the watch for a long time. He turned it over several times and admired it, and then he placed it back into Swami Rama's pocket.

"You don't want it?" Swami Rama asked politely.

"All is God," Swami Vivekananda said sweetly. "There's no difference between you and me, even though we're dressed differently. What difference does it make, then, whose pocket the watch is in?"

Swami Rama was deeply impressed by this and shortly after took his swami vows.

Later Swami Ramathirtha went to America.

No one was sure why he went. He had no plans. He was just intoxicated with love for God. He had only one dhoti wrapped around his neck, nothing else. No warm clothes, no blankets.

He was traveling by sea and one night he was walking out on the deck of the ship. An American gentleman saw him and was attracted to his unusual dress. They began talking and Swami Rama spoke with so much love, as if the two of them had been friends for a thousand years.

"Where are you going, swami?" The man asked.

"To America," Swami Rama replied.

"Which city are you going to?"

"To your city."

"Do you know anyone there?"

"Yes, I know one person."

"And who is that?" The man asked.

"You!" Swami Ramathirtha replied and they both laughed.

Swami Ramathirtha had come to America only to love others.

Try to live a life like this. Just love. Wherever you go, just spread your love. Just keep your candle of love going. Whenever you find a candle unlit, light it up. Get it going, everywhere. There's no other way than that. Remember this principle. Hold on to this principle. All answers lie with love. Suffering is all that's left after losing love.

STORY #42

Lust and the desire for sex are so powerful that even the highest yogis, those who are continuously aware and conscious, are also greatly troubled by it. In the Gita, Lord Krishna says: "The greatest enemy of lust is knowledge. The yogi, the man of knowledge, is trying to destroy it. That's why lust fights so hard with the yogi."

Whenever someone practices yoga, lust takes his entire army and fights against this one yogi. Lust doesn't care about all the other people in the world at that moment. He just wants to defeat the yogi. He tries to catch the yogi. In scientific language, I can explain it this way: There's only one stepladder. You can use it to go up to God, or downward into the senses. Whatever is the source of union with God, is also the source of separation from God.

JAIMINI BATTLES LUST

DURING THE TIME WHEN Lord Vyasa wrote the Bhagavad Gita, he had a powerful disciple named, Jaimini. Since Jaimini was the most advanced disciple of Lord Vyasa, naturally he was an exceptional soul. In fact, Jaimini, himself, is considered to be the author of the Mimamsa System, one of the six classical systems of Indian philosophy.

One day, after Lord Vyasa had finished writing the Gita, he turned to Jaimini and said, "My son. I've completed this work. Please read it over."

Jaimini read the work, but there was one sloka which disturbed him very much. The sloka, written by Lord Vyasa, said, "Even a great yogi, in spite of great effort, can still be drawn into sensual pleasures."

Jaimini couldn't understand this.

"My son," Lord Vyasa said, when he saw Jaimini's puzzled face, "Do you have some doubt about what I've written?"

"Yes, Gurudev," Jaimini said. "You wrote that even a great yogi, in spite of great effort, can still be drawn into sensual pleasures. Then how can we call him a yogi?"

"What you're saying is worth thinking about," Lord Vyasa said. "We'll discuss this tomorrow, as right now I'm quite busy with things."

The great masters often didn't give answers to their disciples right away. They preferred to create situations where their disciples could learn what they needed to learn on their own, and this is what Lord Vyasa decided to.

So he sent Jaimini away for the day.

In the ashram, Lord Vyasa stayed in one hut and Jaimini stayed in another hut. The day ended and nighttime came. That night there was a storm. The sky was covered with clouds. There was lots of lightening and thunder. There was a strong wind. The trees in the woods started moving with great force. It started raining heavily. The animals in the jungle started making noises.

Jaimini was about to go to sleep. Then he heard someone knocking on his door. He was puzzled. Who could be here at night, he asked himself? He heard the knocking again. Then someone called softly.

"Muniji, would you please open the door?"

It was a woman's voice.

He thought to himself, how could there be a woman here at night in the jungle?

But considering there was a storm outside and it was dark, he thought he should open the door. The wind was blowing so heavily that it took a great effort to even open the door. When he did get the door open, the wind caught it and blew it open with great force. At the same moment, lightening flashed.

Standing in front of him was a beautiful young woman with wet clothes. Her beauty was so enchanting that at the same moment as the lightening flashed across the sky, the lightening of lust struck deep in Jaimini's mind.

He thought to himself, I am a yogi. I shouldn't have such a thought in my mind.

But under these circumstances, how could he not give her shelter?

"Muniji," she said sweetly, "It's raining, and there's a bad storm. Would you please let me stay in your hut for the night?"

It was certainly his duty to give her shelter from the storm, but at the same time he recognized his mental condition.

There were two rooms in his hut.

"You may use one of these rooms," he said. "Please go into that room. There're some dry clothes there. Change your clothes and then lock the door and don't open it, even if I ask you to."

What an unusual condition. Just think. What a dangerous condition. The yogi who has been meditating for years and years, and then he comes across such a condition and he falls from all the way up to all the way down.

Don't think that lust is after the yogi in an ordinary way. Lust keeps on testing him. Every minute, he has strong desires. This is such difficult work. There is only one yogi in this world who won't be defeated by lust, by sexual desires. Such an individual is called, the Light of the Universe. My Beloved Gurudev is such a Light of the Universe. He was urduvetta, a master of the sexual energy. Only one who wins the battle with lust can receive the divine body. I consider the divine body most ordinary, but the state of consciousness that it takes you, is worth desiring. Just as after sucking the juice out of the mango, the seed and the skin is useless, so also after attaining to the highest, the body is also useless.

Jaimini had a big storm in his mind. He wasn't an ordinary yogi; he was a great yogi. And his guru was also very high. He was a disciple of a Siddi guru. And he was also a true disciple. So he suffered at seeing his mental condition. When two wrestlers are wrestling and one finds that the other is a little weak, at that moment he puts in extra strength to defeat him. When the Lord of Lust saw that Jaimini was a little weak, he showed tremendous energy. Jaimini saw that just as a big storm was going on outside, so also there was a big storm going on inside his mind.

There was a little hole in the wall of this hut. Jaimini tried to look through it. Isn't this the defeat of a yogi? What an unusual situation. He saw that this woman had taken off all her clothes and was standing naked picking through the dry clothes. Seeing this he lost total control of his mind. He rushed to the door of the room and banged heavily on it.

"Open the door!" He shouted.

The woman inside didn't open the door.

Jaimini became angry. The door was weak, so Jaimini kicked it open. He quickly ran and embraced the naked woman. He gave a strong, lustful hug and closed his eyes and pushed his body against hers.

When he opened his eyes, he saw to his great surprise that the woman had a big beard. It was his own Guru, Lord Vyasa.

Then Vyasa said sweetly,

"My son. Do you still think my sloka is wrong? Aren't you a great yogi?"

Jaimini lowered his eyes. He started crying and fell to his Guru's feet.

These truths of yoga are truly the great truths. It's difficult to even look into this direction of spiritual growth. To walk on it is many more times difficult than that. To remain established in it is even more difficult than that. And to reach to the completion of the journey, the divine body, is almost impossible. There you need the grace of God and Guru.

As long as the Guru doesn't become our leader, our boat won't go to the opposite shore. But don't lose courage listening to this. We have to win the battle, sooner or later. As you gradually and steadily become free of attachments and attractions, you will grow.

My Gurudev taught me a useful technique. It's difficult to use, but it's usable. Men should view older women as their mother, women their own age as their sister, and women younger than them as their daughters. Women should do the same. They should call older men their father, men their own age their brothers, and men younger than them their sons.

But it must come from the depths of your heart and be so piercing and penetrating that it creates the impact of love in the other person.

STORY #43

*There are five scripturally prescribed spiritual disciplines: nonvio-
lence, truth, nonstealing, celibacy, and nonattachment. When any
of these are broken, the mind becomes restless. While a flame in a
windy place flickers unsteadily, a mind in the shelter of these spiritual disciplines burns on steadily. Nonviolence, or ahimsa, is the
first of these disciplines. It means "to not cause distress, in thought,
word, or deed, to any living creature." Its primary position signi-
fies its primary importance. It's the seed of the other four disciplines. When this seed sprouts, truth, nonstealing, celibacy, and
nonattachment manifest spontaneously. The practice of nonviolence
is religion without equal. It's the superb religion for everyone.*

THE SLAVE AND THE LION

ONCE UPON A TIME, there was a slave who desperately
wanted to escape the tortures inflicted by his master. One
dark night he seized his chance to run from his master's
house. When he eventually came to the edge of a large forest, he
was tired by his long run and decided to rest there beneath a large
tree.

"Well," he said to himself, "The forest seems safer than the
city." So, feeling safe, rested, and pleased with himself, he entered
the forest.

He walked for three days, eating only wild fruit. What he
didn't know was that he had chosen a part of the forest that was
inhabited by large, ferocious beasts. Suddenly he heard a lion roar.
His body trembled uncontrollably and his heart raced wildly with
fright.

Turning his eyes skyward, he prayed fervently,

"Oh, Compassionate One! I've struggled hard to free myself
from slavery. I've hardly had a moment to enjoy my freedom, and
now I'm faced with the threat of death. If you desire my death
now, however, I'm prepared to come to you."

The lion roared again. The slave was filled with even more fear when he spotted the lion sitting nearby under a large tree. But curiously enough, the lion didn't seem to be interested in him. The expression on the lion's face even seemed painful. The slave realized, then, that the lion's roar hadn't been the roar of the hunt, but a cry of pain, and the slave's fear subsided.

It seemed that both the lion and the slave were unhappy. They were two individuals in distress whose paths had crossed by chance. Under these circumstances, it is easy for one who is suffering to have sympathy for a fellow-sufferer.

The slave stood up and approached the lion. He saw that one of the lion's hind legs was so infected by a thorn that he couldn't get up. The lion had been roaring from the pain of his wound.

The slave felt great sympathy at the sight of the lion's pain. So he sat beside the lion and looked at the wound. He saw a large thorn deeply embedded in the lion's leg. After gently extracting it, he tossed it into the underbrush. Next he found a small stream. He fashioned a makeshift cup from leaves and filled the cup with water. He gently pressed the wound to squeeze out the pus, and then cleaned it with water. After briefly foraging the forest floor, he found a choice herb which he picked and pounded to a pulp. With this salve, he gently dressed the lion's wound.

The lion was pleased by the slave's tenderness and care. He had sensed from the beginning that this newcomer to the forest was a friend, not an enemy.

During the next two days, the lion and the slave became close friends. The lion could walk with some effort by then, so the slave would lead his limping friend to the stream for a drink. Although the lion had been hungry for three days, his love for the slave had so occupied his mind that he didn't notice his hunger.

A short time later, the wound healed. The lion hunted freely in the woods once again, but each day the lion returned from his hunt to sit beside his friend. Wordlessly and with great affection, the two sat together and gazed into each other's eyes.

Then one day, after about a month of close companionship, the slave decided to try his luck in the city, and the companions parted company reluctantly. As the slave walked away, he looked back at least a dozen times to glimpse his new-found friend sitting at the edge of the forest watching him leave.

The slave entered the city.

In those days a slave without a master could be claimed by anyone. A rich man noticed the slave loitering about and caught him. Fortunately for the slave, however, this new master was a loving man, not mean and cruel like his former master. The slave was immediately grateful for the kind way his new master treated him, so he served his master with love and soon became his favorite slave.

One day the new master heard of a fabulous prize offered to anyone who would dare to wrestle with a ferocious lion that had just been captured in the nearby forest. The master decided to attend the spectacle. Back then it was popular entertainment to watch trained wrestlers fight with fierce animals which had been captured in the forest.

On the day of the event, a large crowd gathered in the arena, including the master and his slave. Everyone was excited because famous wrestlers from all over the kingdom had come to compete for the prize money. Those who had arranged the match, however, had not allowed the wrestlers to see the lion beforehand, and as soon as the ferocious lion was displayed, all the wrestlers refused to compete!

The spectators were disappointed. Then they became angry as no one was brave enough to wrestle the lion. The now desperate sponsors offered, the prize of your choice, to anyone who would wrestle the lion. But still no one came forward.

Then the slave's eyes fell upon the cage of the lion. With a start, he realized that it was his friend pacing in the cage.

"Master," he said to his owner, "I would like to try for the prize, but under two conditions: First, that I'll be able to love the lion, not wrestle with him. And second, that I'll be given the lion itself as my reward if I win."

The master was startled by the slave's strange request, and yet he could see the slave's earnestness. So he approached the sponsors of the event. The sponsors were surprised, but they consented to the slave's conditions.

The angry crowd was already leaving when the sponsors announced,

"Brothers and Sisters! Wait! Although there isn't a wrestler in the house courageous enough to fight this fierce lion, one slave has come forward and has volunteered to try and love him!"

Many spectators laughed. Others were worried for the slave. And when the slave stood up and approached the cage, some speculated that the slave was so fed up with his life that he decided to end it with a daredevil stunt.

The slave approached the cage courageously, and the crowd burst into spontaneous applause and cheers. They held their breath as the slave opened the cage door. They were convinced that as soon as he stepped into the cage, the lion would kill him. They remembered the awful roar of the lion when he was first brought into the arena. It was so loud that several children had fainted. How could such a fierce lion welcome the love of a slave?

As the slave opened the cage door, however, his eyes meet those of the lion. The old friends were delighted to see each other again! The slave entered and gently hugged the lion while the lion affectionately licked his friend's face. The audience was dumbstruck, then enchanted, as if a spell had been cast upon them! No one could fathom this turn of events. Was this a slave or a magician?

Yes, this was truly magic taking place before their very eyes, the magic of love.

The arena was near a small hill outside the city walls. A pathway just beyond the hill led directly to the forest. The slave had decided beforehand to set the lion free, and the sponsors had agreed to his conditions.

"My respected elders," the slave said addressed the crowd. "Please give me your attention. Don't be afraid when I open the cage door and set the lion free. He won't hurt you. My friend and I will quietly walk to the forest. I wish to see him safely home. Six months ago, the hind leg of this lion was infected by a thorn wound. I happened to be in the forest at that time and came upon him. Seeing his pain, I helped heal his wound and we become best friends. I'm not a magician. What I've done didn't come from magic, but from love."

The explanation satisfied the crowd.

The slave reentered the cage and emerged with the lion, but despite the slave's assurances the crowd was still fearful. The lion was so entranced by his savior, however, that he paid no attention to the crowd. Within a few moments, the two friends disappeared behind the hill as the crowd looked on in astonished disbelief.

STORY #44

The Lord teaches in the Shiva Samhita that faith is the first component of any accomplishment. Faith is power itself. The power of mantra, the power in a statue, the power of teacher and teachings, all of these work in proportion to your trust and faith. Whatever amount of faith you have, you will experience that amount of result. As soon as faith is generated in one's mind, progress becomes simple. Sometimes people possess a faith that is not only extraordinary, but miraculous, because their faith is totally different from that of ordinary people.

A CHILD'S FAITH

ONCE UPON A TIME, there was a small village which had received no rain for three years. The inhabitants were totally disheartened. They had tried everything, but nothing had worked.

Their attention, finally, was drawn to their last resort: praying to the Lord.

The residents of this drought-stricken village held a public prayer meeting. This action was taken from helplessness, not from great faith, and half the villagers felt unmotivated to pray.

The meeting time drew near, and crowds of people congregated at the appointed spot. As they waited for prayers to begin, many people chanted bhajans.

A small, ten-year-old orphan boy named, Chapalkumar, entered the tiny house of his poor grandmother. She had cared for him since age seven.

"Grandmother," he said, "I want to go and pray for rain. Where is my umbrella?"

"Your umbrella?" The grandmother replied quizzically.

"Yes," Chapalkumar said.

"Go look near the cupboard."

The boy went to the cupboard.

"Did you find it?" She asked.

"Yes," he said, tucking it under his arm and running quickly out the door.

Along the way, he saw men and women headed in the same direction. Satisfied that he wasn't late, he finally stopped running and began walking with the crowd.

Everyone who saw his umbrella smiled. Many whispered among themselves.

"For the last three years our unfortunate land hasn't had a single drop of rain. There's no sign of rain in sight anywhere. Yet, this boy is carrying an umbrella!"

One man who knew the boy teased him,

"Hey, Chapal!" he said. "Why are you carrying an umbrella?"

"Why shouldn't I?" The boy answered innocently. "We're going to pray to the Lord, so He'll send rain, of course, and we'll all get wet."

Touched by the lad's faith, but still in a teasing manner, the man said,

"Why, of course! Yes, you're right, young man. Why, I ran out of my house in such a hurry that I forgot my umbrella!"

Some people behind them heard the conversation. They joined in the teasing and called out to the man.

"Brother, why are you worried? Don't we have Chapalkumar's umbrella? If it rains, we can all take shelter under it. Chapal, will you allow us to take shelter under your umbrella?"

"Yes, of course," Chapal said, delighted. "But how can we all fit under this small umbrella?"

"Don't worry. We'll find a way," they laughed.

Soon everyone had congregated for prayer at the town square. Those chanting bhajans stopped. A well-known gentleman of the city stood up and in sorrowful tones, described the drought situation. Then after praising the greatness of the Compassionate Lord, he explained the importance of prayers. He concluded with a humble plea:

"Dearest brothers and sisters, let us pray silently to the Lord with pure hearts for just two minutes."

After the silent prayer, he prayed out loud, calling to the Lord in a humble voice:

"Oh, Compassionate One, bring us rain! Oh, Compassionate One, bring us rain! Oh, Compassionate One, bring us rain!"

No one believed the prayers would work, but no sooner had the people begun their heartfelt prayers, than a sudden flash of lightening snapped across the sky. There was a sharp clap of thunder and the wind blew fiercely. Within moments, the sky filled with dense clouds and everyone's eyes filled with tears. Their prayers had come to life.

Everyone chanted a bhajan with deep emotion to conclude the assembly and by the time they left, rain was pouring down in torrents.

Chapalkumar danced ecstatically. Unfolding his umbrella, he invited everyone to come under it.

"Come! Come! Come under my umbrella!" He called.

A man lifted Chapalkumar up onto his shoulders, and the entire crowd walked as if each person were covered by the umbrella.

Was Chapal's umbrella just an umbrella, then?

STORY #45

Service without love isn't service, and service with love is more
than service. One who sees faults in others can't progress on the
spiritual path. One who sees the master's vices, rather than his
virtues, can't absorb the essence of service. Since the master is only
human, he will naturally commit mistakes. A fine quality servant,
however, considers his master to be everything in life. If the
servant does anything to displease the master, the servant shouldn't
try to prove that the master's order was mistaken. Instead, he
should regret having misunderstood his master's intentions. Thus,
the temperament of a vigilant servant should dispose him to see his
own faults and to remove them. After all, a mad person doesn't find
fault with his head when his leg slips into a ditch.

THE FAITHFUL SERVANT

ONCE UPON A TIME, an intelligent King was seeking a personal servant. Through his state attendants, he publicly
advertised this post and arranged to spend an entire day
interviewing candidates. On the appointed day, approximately
one hundred hopeful candidates came, and the State Attendant
informed the King the candidates were waiting.

"Send them in one by one," The King ordered.

The first applicant entered the room, greeted the King, and
then stood politely waiting for instructions.

"There's a pot of water sitting on the table in front of you," the
King said. "Next to it are some glasses. Bring me a glass filled
with water."

"As you wish, Your Majesty," the man said, and he brought
the King a glass of water.

Then the King gave him a second order.

"Now throw this glass away in the bathroom."

"As you wish, Your Majesty," the man said, obeying the order
without hesitation.

When the applicant returned to the King, however, the King scolded him.

"Why did you throw that glass away?" The King asked.

"Because you ordered me to do so, Your Majesty," the baffled applicant replied.

The King silently pointed to the door and the applicant left feeling confused and dejected.

One by one, the other applicants came before the King.

The King gave the same order to each applicant: to fetch water in a glass and then to throw the glass away in the bathroom. Afterwards, the King asked the same question.

"Why did you throw that glass away?"

Each applicant gave the same answer.

"Because you ordered me to do so, Your Majesty."

Each time the King pointed silently to the door. Not a single person passed the test.

There was one applicant, however, who had arrived first and was sitting patiently and comfortably in the corner. When the state servant gave him a chance to see the King, this applicant politely replied,

"I'll go last. I'm in no hurry."

One by one, the other applicants continued to fail the test. Invariable the applicants still waiting to see the King, would ask in a worried voice,

"Brother, are you finished? What does the King want you to do?"

Everyone said the same thing.

"First the King ordered me to bring him a glass of water. Then he told me to throw it away in the bathroom. After I did that, he scolded me and asked me why I threw away the glass of water. And I replied, 'Because you ordered me to do it.' What else could I have possibly said?"

Finally, it was time for the last applicant, the one who had arrived first, to take his turn. He went to the King, bowed to him with tears in his eyes, and knelt down humbly at his feet. In a voice choked with emotion, he said,

"Oh, Master of the Earth, I've been wanting to see you so badly. For a long time, I've fervently cherished the wish to serve you. And, now, the gracious Lord has finally fulfilled my desire and has given me my first chance to do so."

On hearing his sweet and affectionate speech, the King was pleased, but he gave no outward sign of this. Instead, he gave the applicant the same order: "Go and bring me a glass of water."

The applicant eagerly complied.

"Now, throw it away in the bathroom."

The applicant threw the glass on the bathroom floor. The glass broke and water splashed all over.

"Why did you spill that water?" the King scolded. "Why did you break that glass?"

"Oh, most gracious one!" The applicant said, immediately bowing and folding his hands and speaking in a humbly voice, "I've committed a mistake. Please forgive me. I'll never repeat it again."

This applicant didn't say: "Because you told me so," as the others had done. Their replies were merely intended to defend themselves and had clearly shown the King that they believed the King was at fault, and not themselves.

The King was extremely impressed with this applicant's attitude. Thus, he employed the man on the spot. Although the ninety-nine other applicants had come with the hope of serving the King, they had no interest in the King's needs; they were only concerned with the glamour of the job. The last applicant, however, hadn't come for a fancy job; he had come to serve. His sole concern was for the King's welfare, rather than fulfilling his own fantasies about the position.

Story #46

Self observation without judgement is essential for spiritual growth. We must be patient. Each night we should review our day and learn from it, and treat ourselves with great love. When workers spread fresh cement on the floor you can't walk on it for two or three days. If you walk on it before it's ready, you'll leave footprints forever. And so it is on the spiritual path, some things take time.

A Saint Hurts My Feelings

ONCE I WENT FOR the darshan of a very old and famous Mahatma in India. He was traveling by train and I heard that his train was going to make a short stop in the town where I lived. He had many disciples in my town and they, too, wanted to see him.

I was a swami by then, but I was a young swami. The social custom in India is that saints should always be pleased to see each other, and the older saint should be garlanded by the younger saint.

The train stopped and Mahatma Guruji came out and stood in the doorway of the train car so everybody could have his darshan. Hundreds of people pressed close to see him. I applied sandalwood to his forehead and placed a garland around his neck and he smiled at me. Normally in India when an older saint greets a younger saint, the older saint will embrace the younger saint. He won't just smile; he'll take a special moment and embrace the younger saint. They do this to encourage the younger saint.

On this particular day, Mahatma Guruji just smiled at me. He smiled sweetly, but he didn't embrace me and I was a little bit hurt.

The train left and I returned to my residence. I thought deeply about what had happened. Then I realized that it was impossible for him to embrace me. There were hundreds of people pressing close for his blessing. Furthermore, he was standing two steps above me and he was much older than me and it would have been difficult for him to bend over that far and embrace me without causing pain to his body.

So I realized my expectation was incorrect, not the action of Mahatma Guruji, and I became happy. I had figured out truly what had happened and I was no longer hurt.

The next day, to my great surprise, I received a visit. Mahatma Guruji's main disciple came to see me. He was a wealthy land-owner and he traveled with Mahatma Guruji to take care of his needs. He had come to my residence only to pay his respects to me.

"After our train left your town," he told me, "Gurudev talked about you and he praised you over and over and he sent me to see you. He loves you very much."

There is a phrase in India: I recognized my mistake and I held my own hand. It means: I took responsibility for my own wrong thought or action.

This is the essence of the story. This is what we should re-member from this story.

I saw Mahatma Guruji one more time. Several years passed. Accidently he fell on the bank of the Nirmada River and hurt his leg badly. They brought him to Daboine for medical care. By chance, I was staying only 10 miles away. It was Guru Purnima, so he had his Guru Purnima in Daboine and I went for his darshan one more time before he died.

STORY #47

*The spiritual history of India is so great that it's almost beyond de-
scription. Even now, in India's sad state, there are still samskaras,
or impressions, from this past glory. One of these customs is that
a person may adopt the clothes of a swami and be taken care of by
society. Today in India there are hundreds of thousands of sadhus
and they are all fed, clothed, and housed by Indian society, even by
the poorest of the poor.*

*Naturally, some abuse this system. But India believes that
saints are the gems of the country and just as it takes tons of coal
to produce one diamond, it takes tons of sadhus to produce one true
saint. India believes this is worthwhile. One sun in the sky is
enough. It's enough for the entire world.*

NARSINH MAHETA AND THE BANK DRAFT

NARSINH MAHETA WAS ONE such great soul. He isn't
known here in America, so I want to tell you about him.
I'll tell you a little about his life and then I'll tell you a
popular story about him.

He lived about 1200 years ago in my home state of Gujarat and
he was a great devotional poet. Even today his devotional songs
are sung all over Gujarat. The use of the word bhakta or devotional person isn't appropriate for him, because this word describes
an ordinary devotee. Narsinh Maheta was a true yogi and so we
refer to him as a bhakta yogi.

Although he was married and followed the path of a householder, he was still a perfect sanyasi. Although he lived in the city,
he was still a yogi. This is because of his knowledge of the oneness
of all things. To him there was no difference between the city and
the forest, between the life of a sanyasi and that of a householder.

He had a wife and two children. His home was like a temple. In
one room disciples and guests chanted constantly and sang dhuns
and bhajans to God. He had Indian instruments for them, drums,

cymbals, and a tamboura, so devotees could sing. In another room, devotees read scripture and chanted japa.

He saved no money, but his popularity was such that guests arrived daily for his darshan and offered gifts at his holy feet. These gifts he never considered as his own, but as gifts in service to the great saints. This is how he passed his whole life.

One day two pilgrims arrived in his town. They were on their way to Dwaraka to visit the Krishna temples. They were making their pilgrimage on foot and they didn't know which road to take to Dwaraka. They had to pass through a forest and they were afraid of being robbed. There were no banks back then and they were carrying 700 rupees, which was a lot of money.

Narsinh Maheta lived in Junagadh. It was a large city and still is, and the pilgrims wanted to find a rich man who would take their money and then write them a note, like a check, which they could cash in Dwaraka with another rich man. That way if they were robbed, they wouldn't lose their money.

The pilgrims entered the Junagadh town square. A group of young people were sitting around talking and having fun. That was the purpose of the town square. People gathered there to socialize and have fun, especially in the evening. The young people saw the two pilgrims and decided to have some fun with them.

"Jai Shri Krishna!" They all said sarcastically when the pilgrims approached, and they put their hands together in the prayer position.

"Jai Shri Krishna!" The pilgrims said with joy. They thought it was wonderful to meet such a saintly group of young people.

"Where are you going?" They asked.

"We're going to Dwaraka," the pilgrims said, "and we need a note from a rich person. We're carrying some money for our trip and we're afraid of being robbed. Please give us the address of a rich person."

"Oh, there're lots of rich people here in Junagadh!" the young people said, but there's one special one," and they whispered among themselves. "Come with us. We'll take you to his home. That way you won't get lost."

"How kind of you!" the pilgrims said.

"Oh, it's not a question of kindness!" the young people said. "It's our sevadharma, our service to God's children! It's our holy karma!" They laughed to themselves as they said this.

They led the two pilgrims through the streets of Junagadh.

"But one thing you should know," they said as they walked. "This rich man doesn't like people to know that he's rich. So at first he may say:

I'm not a rich man. I'm poor. I'm a devotee of God. I don't have any money, not a single rupee. Somebody has deceived you. Somebody is making fun of you, and me. No rich people in Dwaraka know me. Who would I address this note to?

But don't believe him when he talks like this! He says this to everyone! He dresses like a saint and he doesn't live in a big mansion, but he has lots of money."

"What's his name?" The pilgrims asked.

"Narsinh Maheta," the young people replied, and they could hardly keep from laughing.

They knew Narsinh had no money at all, nothing.

When the group arrived at Narsinh Maheta's house, they stopped a short distance away and pointed to his house and then they left. They slapped their hands together and burst into laughter.

Narsinh Maheta received the pilgrims with love and listened to their story and insisted that the pilgrims stay with him for two days to rest. Then he told them as they were leaving,

"But dear friends, I'm a poor man. I don't have any money. I'm only a devotee of God. No rich person knows me in Dwaraka. Please find someone else in Junagadh to write you a note."

The pilgrims were ready for these words and they insisted with great firmness,

"No! We'll accept a note only from you! You have a saintly character and we trust you!"

Narsinh Maheta now knew for certain that someone was playing a trick on them. He left immediately for his meditation room and sat at the feet of the Holy Lord.

"Beloved Krishna," he prayed. "I'm a dull man, a simple devotee. I don't understand You're divine play. The only person in

Dwaraka who knows me is You. I can write a note for these pilgrims on Your name only. Please accept this note. If you don't, these sincere pilgrims may be robbed. Please give me the command and I'll write a note for them on Your name"

"Write!" Lord Krishna said.

"Which one of Your Holy names should I use?" Narsinh Maheta asked.

"Shamala Seth," Lord Krishna said.

And so Narsinh Maheta wrote a note that said:

Shamala Seth, Beloved Almighty Lord Krishna, kindly pay 700 hundred rupees to the pilgrims carrying this note. Your humble servant, Narsinh Maheta. I pranam again and again to You with great love.

The pilgrims left and by chance they met the same group of young people who had played the trick on them.

"Were you comfortable in the home of Narsinh Maheta?" They asked with a twinkle in their eyes.

"Oh, yes!" They both said together. "He's a divine man!"

"And did you get your note?"

"Yes, but at first he refused strongly just like you said."

"Whose name did he use in Dwaraka?" They asked.

"Shamala Seth," the pilgrims replied.

Later that evening when the young men were alone in the town square, one said,

"I lived for 5 years in Dwaraka. I don't remember any rich man with that name."

"Narsinh Mareta is such a sweet talker! What do you think he'll do with the 700 rupees?"

"Who knows. He'll spoil the name of Junagadh for everyone now."

The two pilgrims arrived safely in Dwaraka. They visited all the famous places and prayed in the temples. They were extremely happy and totally pleased with their trip. Then it was time to cash their note. They asked all over, but no one had heard of Shamala Seth. They looked for three days and finally people said they had been cheated by someone in Junagadh.

"No, that's impossible," they said.

On the fourth day, they met some horsemen on a road. Behind them was a recluse billionaire riding in an ornate gold-plated chariot. The people of Dwaraka knew of his existence, but seldom saw him. His name was Krishna Mohan.

"We're visiting Dwaraka," one of the pilgrims said. "May we have a moment with Mohanji?"

"Bring the pilgrims to me!" The rich man called. "Tell me your story in my castle where it's more comfortable."

The pilgrims described their whole journey to the rich man and then they showed him the note. The eyes of the rich man filled with tears.

"Everyone in Dwaraka knows me as Krishna Mohan, but my parents call me Shamala, and I like that name very much. It's a name of great affection and only those who truly love me call me by that name. I'll honor your note."

Back in Junagadh, poor Narsinh Maheta had been praying for many days, ever since he had written the note, begging for forgiveness.

"Forgive me, Lord. Forgive me, Lord. I've taken 700 rupees from two pure pilgrims."

"Narsinh!" Lord Krishna replied, "Don't you think I have 700 rupees! If you had asked for 700,000 rupees, I would have given you that!"

The deeper meaning of this story is that when the devotee becomes one with God through devotion, God works through the devotee. And so it was God who had written the note, not Narsinh Maheta.

STORY #48

Satsang means to sit in the company of truth. In satsang we purify our minds and increase our devotion through contact with a saint or other truth seekers. At that time we should relax our mind and give up our worldly thoughts and gradually our mental impurities will be washed away.

THE RICH FARMER'S FIRST TRAIN RIDE

A LONG TIME AGO the train was new in India. At first people were afraid of it. There used to be more people just standing there watching the train than there were using it. They were afraid that if the train overturned, they would die.

So in each railroad station the employees used to treat the few passengers with great care. They used to stand and greet everyone and help them to their seats. Gradually people got used to trains, until today in India people rush and push to get seats and even ride on top of the cars where for sure they would get hurt if anything happened.

In those early days there was one rich farmer who decided to go to Bombay. He packed his things and dressed in fresh clothes and went to the train station. He waited patiently awhile in the train station and watched the other passengers. They were all dressed so nicely and were smiling and saying good-by to their loved ones.

The train station was large and there was more than one train. There were five or six trains all waiting to leave at different times. He picked out the best one, the one he thought was the most beautiful, and sat on that one. This was his first train ride and he wanted to ride on the best train.

But he never checked where the train was going. He just selected it because he liked the way it looked.

The train left the station. After a short time a friendly man sitting next to him asked,

"Where are you going?"

"I'm going to Bombay," the rich farmer replied.

"Bombay?" The man said, "But this train is going to Ahmedabad. Bombay is the other way."

"That's alright," the rich farmer said. "Let it go to Ahmedabad."

"But sir! You said you wanted to go to Bombay. You're going in the wrong direction. You're going to Ahmedabad."

The rich farmer took out his ticket and showed it to the man.

"My ticket says Bombay," he said. "Doesn't this driver know that? Doesn't he know I have a ticket for Bombay? That's his mistake. Why isn't this train going to Bombay?"

Sometimes we're all like this rich farmer. We come rich in thoughts to satsang and can't change the tracks in our mind and catch the train of devotion to God.

STORY #49

Even saints can be classified as high, medium, or ordinary. The story I'll tell you now is about a medium caliber saint. This saint, however, was the best of the medium caliber saints as he was learning to master nonattachment. He never stayed anywhere for more than two or three days, nor did he ever choose the direction of his travel. He simply moved wherever his feet took him.

THE LONG-HAIRED SAINT AND THE WIND

ONE MORNING LATURIA MAHARAJ was walking on the road. He gave no thought at all to where he was headed. The wind was blowing fiercely against his back and his long hair kept blowing in his face. He had to repeatedly brush his hair away from his face with his hands, but to no avail.

Finally, he reached the limit of his patience. He abruptly turned around and spoke to the strong wind with fire in his eyes and told the wind to leave him alone, but the wind ignored him. He began to walk again in the same direction, but the wind once again rudely blew Laturia's hair in his face. He turned around a second time and ordered the wind to stop, but the wind ignored him completely. Exasperated, he stopped again and muttered to himself,

"This silly wind is causing mischief today. I'll have to figure this problem out or it will continue to bother me for the rest of the day."

So, Laturia Maharaj turned around and started walking in the opposite direction, directly into the wind. With a triumphant smile on his face, he said,

"Hello, my friend! Now do your mischief!"

The wind now blew his hair behind him, away from his face and the rest of his day went well.

When we move in the direction of attachment, our desires, the wind in this story, constantly bothers us. One desire leads to another. Our peace of mind, the hair in this story, is constantly disturbed. When we change directions and move toward nonattachment and a simplier life, our lives become more peaceful.

STORY #50

> As long as we simply listen to spiritual teachings or read about
> them, we'll grow little. Certainly in the beginning it's important to
> listen, but then we must reflect, absorb the principle, and apply it
> to our lives. If we don't change one wrong quality or add one new
> good quality, what's the use of going further in our spiritual work?
> That's why in ancient India the great rishis gave short discourses.

ARJUNA'S OLDEST BROTHER

IN THE BHAGAVAD GITA, Arjuna was Lord Krishna's most
beloved disciple. Arjuna had four brothers. The oldest was
Yudhishthir. In Sanscrit his name is beautiful. It means:
One who remains steady in war. Here war means the war we all
have to fight to recapture our own soul bliss.

Yudhishthir had all the desirable divine qualities of a true sadhak. He always spoke the truth. He observed the dharma properly
and for this reason he was later called, Dharmaraj: the master of
religion, the master of duty.

This is a story about his childhood.

There were five brothers in all and one hundred uncles. They
ruled India, so the brothers were all princes and given a special education. When the brothers were young, they all studied together.
They had one teacher who was especially strict. One day when
Yudhishthir was still a child, this teacher noticed that he was still
reading the very first lesson. The other brothers had completed
lesson twenty and the teacher got angry.

"Why are you still reading this lesson?" He demanded. "You're
the oldest and yet the others have passed you!"

Yudhishthir didn't reply, but simply kept reading the first
lesson.

Three or four times this happened and yet Yudhishthir didn't
put the first lesson down. Finally, his teacher slapped him hard on
the cheek.

"What is it that you don't understand?" He demanded.

Yudhishthir became very humble.

"Guruji," he said. "I know how to read all the other lessons my brothers have finished. But here in lesson one it is written: Don't be angry, and I can't do that yet."

Then his teacher calmed down and realized that he, too, was still on the first lesson.

STORY #51

*We can undertake and complete several vocations in our life.
However, the attainment of God is so difficult that even if one puts
all his effort and concentration into the task, he may not succeed in
a lifetime. The seeker who wishes to attain God should close the
gates to all activities and keep open only the gate to the Lord. To
attempt to attain the Lord Almighty means to sacrifice one's whole
life to this holy cause. To make a garland, we bind together flowers
on a string. The seeker must sacrifice his soul, tie all his actions on
the thread of God, and be hit by Cupid's arrow in his love for God,
or he can't be an upashak and make real progress. Sadhana takes
great patience. When I first started my deeper sadhana, I thought I
would be finished in six months.*

LORD BUDDHA LEARNS FROM A SQUIRREL

LORD BUDDHA WAS DEPRESSED. He had been performing a difficult yoga sadhana for many years without finding confirmation of his experience in the yogic scriptures. His faith was wavering and his enthusiasm for practice had subsided. He wasn't interested in anything.

"I was foolish to give up my royal luxuries for the lifestyle of a sanyasi," he thought.

His depression lasted for days. Finally he decided to leave sanyas and return to the city of Kapilvastu. The next morning he woke up and ate, but didn't do his yoga sadhana. Then he bathed, dressed, and set forth for Kapilvastu.

At noon, Lord Buddha entered a village where he begged for food. After obtaining a meager meal, he sat down to eat on the bank of a lake on the outskirts of the village. Exhausted by his state of depression, he stretched out to relax under the shade of a large tree.

Then he spotted a squirrel who repeatedly dipped her tail into the lake, ran a short distance away, and then shook the water off.

Lord Buddha watched the squirrel for awhile and then his curiosity was aroused. He approached the squirrel and asked,

"Sister, what are you doing?"

"I want to empty this lake," the squirrel replied in a firm voice.

"But, sister," Lord Buddha said, "How many lifetimes will it take you, a small squirrel to empty this lake? Why do you want to do that?"

"My child has drowned in this lake," the squirrel said.

Pity flowed from Lord Buddha's heart into his voice.

"But Little Sister," he said tenderly, "You won't be able to finish this task in a thousand lifetimes."

"I don't care!" the squirrel said. "I'm not concerned with whether I finish or not. I'll continue to make an effort. Let it be a thousand lifetimes or a million lifetimes. A decision is a decision! You're an ascetic and a holy man. Please bless me so that my determination doesn't waver."

Gazing compassionately upon the small squirrel, Lord Buddha blessed her. Then he bowed reverently to her and returned to sit under the shade of the tree.

"My own determination is so weak compared to that of the squirrel," he said to himself in disgust. "There's no comparison. Even though the squirrel's determination is charged with anger at the lake and mine is charged with love for the Lord, I'm inspired by her example and I'll persevere with my original decision. From now on I'll courageously confront all situations I encounter until I reach the summit of my sadhana and accomplish samadhi."

This decision destroyed his deep depression. Lack of faith scurried swiftly from his mind. Determination returned. His enthusiasm was revived. With a firm step and with a revival of interest in life, Lord Buddha got up and returned to his place of sadhana.

"I'll accomplish samadhi, or I'll die," he said, and every fiber of his body was filled with conviction

If only ordinary effort, patience, power, and knowledge are brought to a task, then the results will be ordinary. The tasks taken up by great men call for extraordinary effort, patience, power, and knowledge. The necessary virtues are confidence, knowledge, unrelenting effort, deep faith, great fondness for the task at hand, and patience.

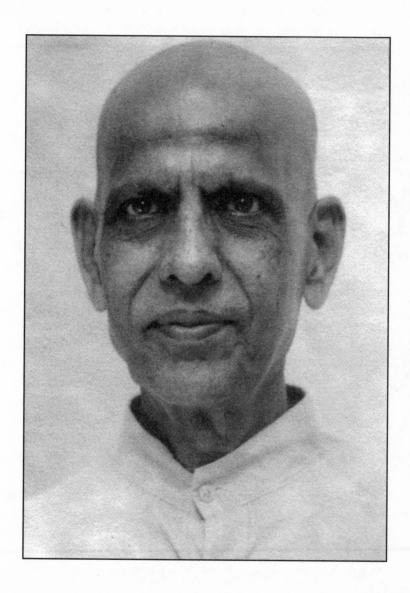

STORY #52

Compassion is born when we can feel the pain of others. We all have our own pains to suffer, but those who suffer for the pain of others are especially loved by God. Just think, we all can become great philanthropists. We can all give comfort to the hearts of others by giving a loving glance to someone in despair, or by addressing an afflicted person as Brother or Sister.

SIDDHARTHA SAVES A SWAN

ONCE UPON A TIME many guests came to the palace of Siddhartha's father, King Shuddhodan, to celebrate an important occasion. Many princes of small and large kingdoms came for the occasion.

In those days men of the warrior caste were taught the martial arts starting in early childhood.

In one part of the garden, some young princes between ten and twelve years old were practicing archery. A flock of swans flew low overhead, barely thirty or forty feet from the ground. The princes shouted with joy and took aim at the birds. The arrow of one prince pierced a swan and sent it spiraling to the ground.

Young Siddhartha was playing with his friends in the same garden. He saw the flock of swans, too, and he was watching when the swan fell to the ground. From early childhood, he had been loving and compassionate, so his tender heart felt a stab of pain when he saw the swan fall.

Quickly he ran to the spot where the swan had fallen. He examined the bird and determined the wound was superficial. Very tenderly, being careful not to prevent further injury, he removed the arrow.

Meanwhile, the young prince who had shot the arrow arrived and gloated,

"That's my swan! I shot it!"

"No!" Siddhartha said firmly, "The swan is mine! The swan belongs to its savior, not to its destroyer. I saved the swan by pulling out the arrow and now I'll nurse it back to health."

They argued heatedly. Neither boy would change his mind.

Then an elderly man approached. He had been sitting nearby listening attentively to their conversation. When he spoke, both boys knew, his word was final.

"Only the savior can be the master," he said. "The swan belongs to Siddhartha because he saved the swan's life."

The hunter prince left still angry.

For the next month, Siddhartha stayed with the swan. He stopped attending palace festivals because he was too busy feeding, watering and caring for the bird.

At the end of a month, the swan was completely healed and could fly on its own again. Siddhartha took the beautiful bird into the wild and set it free. When he saw the swan flying fast and high in the open blue sky, free and healthy again, his heart was full of joy.

STORY #53

Character building is necessary for life to flourish. It can be built best with the bricks of yama and niyama. One of these practices is arjava, or straightforwardness, which means 'simplicity, or purity of the body, the organs, and the mind.' When we practice purity of the body we're concerned with using our body only for worthy actions. When we practice purity of the sense organs, we're concerned only with sights worth seeing, words worth hearing, and smells worth smelling. When we practice purity of mind, we contemplate only those thoughts which are simple and innocent and determine never to deceive anyone. Sometimes, though, even innocent people deceive us, but their deception is motivated by love, not selfishness. This is a story of innocent deception.

THE SCULPTOR AND HIS SON

ONCE UPON A TIME there was a well-known sculptor named, Ratneshwar. He wanted his son, Davarashmi, to follow in his footsteps and to surpass his achievements, as well. With this aim in mind, Ratneshwar guided his son's effort from early childhood. As a result, Devarashmi became a devoted student of sculpture.

Since Ratneshwar was as skilled at teaching as he was at sculpting, he was able to teach his son many advanced techniques as well as to keep him highly inspired. And since Devarashmi was a keen student, Ratneshwar and Devarashmi complemented one another and made a good father and son team.

At the early age of twenty, Devarashmi's sculptures were respected all over India and he became one of the highest ranking sculptors in the country. Whenever his works were praised, Devarashmi would run happily to his father to share his joy with him.

"This famous artist has highly praised my sculpture!" Devarashmi would say. Or, "This sculpture is one of my best pieces!"

Ratneshwar would pat his son's head affectionately. Then he would give him the same speech.

"Yes," he would say, "I also like this work. However, it's not your best piece of art, although I like it very much. You're still young. To understand the secret of art you must practice for many more years. Every great artist in his early years felt just as you do now. But as they matured and went deeper into their work, they realized that a work they once considered to be their best, was really quite ordinary. It's only after creating many pieces that the artist attains the vitality and subtlety of his art. Artistic excellence develops gradually. If a genuine artist was asked on his deathbed, "Which of your works do you considered to be your best?" He would reply with grief:

"My dear brother, my best piece of work remains in my imagination. During my life I struggled hard to create my masterpiece, but everything I've created so far has captured only a part of what I've visualized. My most recent work merely captures what I most recently see, but I don't consider it to be my best piece of art."

Devarashmi didn't like to hear this. He especially didn't like his father's analysis of his work. He believed that his father hadn't carefully evaluated his work.

One day he told his father,

"You haven't evaluated my art in the manner that the famous artists at the gallery have."

Ratneshwar understood his son's feelings. He knew the value of encouragement, yet he also understood that praise generated pride and pride blocked the development of the artist by clouding his creative faculty. He also believed that when evaluating a work of art, one should praise its good features in the beginning and its flaws at the end. And furthermore, the artist should take no offense, for when a critic gives constructive criticism, his aim is to help the artist improve. His comments shouldn't be taken as blame or negativity.

Devarashmi, though, felt hurt. He was certain his father's evaluation of his sculpture didn't measure up to the praise of the other artists.

Ratneshwar understood this, also.

"The artists who praised your work are older, highly experienced lovers of sculpture," he said. "They see you as a budding artist in need of inspiration through praise."

But Devarashmi still wasn't satisfied and disagreements of this type continued to occur between him and his father. Eventually, Devarashmi became convinced that his father wasn't properly evaluating his art. He wanted his father to respect his art as being superior, not just ordinary.

Devarashmi continued to work hard and often placed his new pieces in his father's hands, asking for critical analysis of the flaws.

Ratneshwar was well acquainted with his son's nature, so he deliberately avoided pointing out faults in his work.

"My son," he would say, hoping his son would find and remove his own faults,

"You're an artist of the new generation and I belong to the old generation. We have different tastes. What I see as a weakness, you may see as a strength. From my viewpoint, I definitely see faults in your work. However, I want you to find them yourself."

The father, though, knew his son still needed guidance. So one day Ratneshwar found an indirect way to counsel his son. He selected a piece of sculpture by an artist who had faults similar to his son's, and he discussed those faults with Devarashmi.

When Devarashmi saw his own shortcomings reflected in the works of other artists, he found it easier to admit to them. Sometimes he would say,

"Father, I made that same mistake in the sculpture I just created."

"Please bring me your sculpture," his father would reply.

Devarashmi would then bring the sculpture and point out the flaws, himself, to his father.

This is the method Ratneshwar used to correct his son's mistakes.

One day one of Devarashmi's sculptures won first prize in an exhibition. As usual, his father didn't agree with the critic's praise and Devarashmi was frustrated once more with his father's opinion.

This time Devarashmi was convinced that his father was praising his work to other artists, but was concealing the praise from him. So he decided to force his father to reveal his true opinion.

He devised a plan.

He began secretly working on a new piece of sculpture. His intention was to present the finished piece as that of another artist from the same school of thought as his own. Then he would engage his father in a discussion on the merits, or demerits, of the work.

As Devarashmi worked in secret, he also initiated conversations with his father on the most subtle nuances of technique and he employed these techniques in his secret project. Ratneshwar was delighted to witness his son's sharp mind. With joy and affection he spoke with his son about the art of sculpture, subtle techniques in design, and blessed his son saying,

"You're going to be the best sculptor in all of India."

When his secret sculpture was finished, Devarashmi traveled 500 miles to the site of an ancient cultural center where archeologists were on a dig. Taking the sculpture that he had worked on so carefully, he rubbed it with dirt and buried it where the archeologists were sure to find it.

Six months later the newspapers were full of praise for what was described as an ancient work of art found at this site. Someone drew Ratneshwar's attention to it and he read all the various articles and published descriptions about the find. Moved by the beautiful pictures of the ancient work of art, he told his son, "Devarashmi, let's travel to this cultural center. We'll see and learn many things there."

Devarashmi agreed.

On reaching their destination, father and son saw crowds of people. Throngs had been coming daily to see the newly excavated statues. Since both father and son were well-known sculptors, the organizers respectfully welcomed them and courteously gave them all the information about the excavations. Guides showed them the various sites and ancient remains.

Finally they were shown the unique piece of art which had just been excavated.

After inspecting it carefully, Ratneshwar exclaimed,

"Devarashmi, this is the best and most unique piece of sculpture that I've ever seen, ancient or modern. I see in this work certain concepts that I, myself, have been trying to express, but so far have been only able to imagine. This piece looks as if a skilled artist has found a beautiful balance between ancient and modern art. It also appears to be a beautiful mixture of contemporary and future art, as well. This is the path which I'm trying to lead you."

The tour guide left for a moment and father and son stood alone.

Devarashmi lifted the statue, turned it upside down, and showed it to his father. Written on the bottom was the name,

"Devarashmi."

Ratneshwar's eyes filled with tears of joy.

"My son," he said. "By not excessively praising your work, I was trying to prevent you from becoming egotistical. Art is like an ocean and the artist is like a drop. No matter how skilled and how great an artist may be, he'll always fail to accommodate the ocean of possibilities in the droplet of his intellect. Art isn't intended for competition, awards, or greed. Art created for these purposes is materialistic, rather than artistic. True art involves creating something for the sake of creation. In that is found divine joy, the artist's true reward."

Devarashmi was touched by his father's pure heart and high ideals. Bowing down, he touched his father's feet and asked for his blessing.

"I'm your son," he said. "But please bless me that I may become your disciple and embody your principles and virtues in my life."

Embracing his son, Ratneshwar said,

"My son, you yourself are my best piece of art. Although I love all my sculptures, I love you much more, for they're inert and you're living. You have my life and you're my best creation.

You already are my disciple. You have my blessing. Continue to progress in your art."

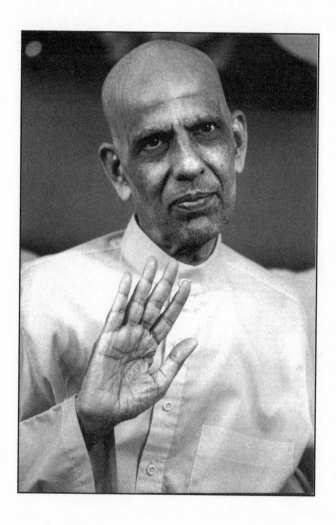

STORY #54

We begin to recognize our own individual existence a few years after birth. The moment we begin to distinguish between yours and mine, attachment is born. In Sanscrit, the word is parigraha and it means 'to store or accumulate with strong attachment,' or 'to cling firmly to,' or 'to fasten completely to.' Nonattachment is a virtue because it creates a peaceful mind. A person practicing non-attachment cultivates voluntary simplicity and discharges his or her duties in life while remaining free of obsessive desires.

THE SAINT AND THE DIRT PILE

ONE DAY A RENUNCIANT saint came to a large city. He noticed that a concrete road had been built beside a dusty dirt road. An old, broken bamboo basket lay beside the dirt road. He picked the basket up and began filling it with dirt and emptying it onto the concrete road. After a few hours, he had a huge mound of dirt on the concrete road.

Anyone watching his actions would have considered him crazy, and crazy he was. But his madness was from practicing yoga, rather than from mental disorder. He was suffering from the madness of love and devotion. He was a yoga seeker, but he had been led astray.

Later that afternoon the renunciant saint finished making an enormous pile of dirt right in the middle of the concrete road. Then he sat in the lotus position on top of the pile as if he had worked all those hours just to sit there like that.

Just then the king's procession came down the same road. Usually the roads on which the king's procession traveled were decided in advance so that the state officers could prepare the way. But today the king had changed his mind and had taken this new road.

As the king's attendants rode ahead to clear the road, they saw the large pile of dirt in the middle of the road with an apparently crazy person sitting on top. Since they couldn't clear the way in time for the king to pass, the only thing they could do was ask the 'mad person' sitting there to move. The chief horseman looked at the man and concluded he was a saint. Since everyone knew that the king was religious and never ridiculed any saint, the chief horseman approached the saint and humbly said,

"The king is coming."

The saint gazed indifferently at the attendant.

"Who?" He yawned.

"The king of the city," replied the horseman.

"Let him come," the saint said. "There's enough room for him to pass."

"But he's the king," the horseman persisted. "He shouldn't have to suffer the humiliation of squeezing past one of his subjects. You should get up and move."

"Me, get up? Why should I get up?" Quibbled the saint. "If there's a king coming then I'm entitled to remain here. I'm an emperor! There's plenty of room for him to pass by."

It wasn't possible to remove the saint from the dirt pile without using force and the king had ordered long ago that nobody should be harassed during his processions. So the horseman returned to the king and explained,

"Your Highness! There's a saint sitting on top of a dirt pile in the middle of the road. When I told him to get up he said, 'I'm not moving. I'm an emperor. The king has plenty of room to pass by if he wants.'"

The king smiled.

"All right," he said. "It's fine. We'll pass by."

The procession continued. When they came to the saint, the king halted the procession and came down from on atop his elephant. Approaching the saint, he offered pranams and humbly asked,

"Are you really an emperor?"

"Yes," replied the saint. "There's no doubt about it."

"What's the difference between a king and an emperor?" The king asked.

"A king is a prisoner of a small or large state," the saint said. "He isn't free to leave his state or his palace and live in another state. He can't travel alone. Twenty-five to fifty people have to carry him from one place to another. I'm an emperor. I can move about in any state whenever I want unaccompanied by anyone."

The king was pleased with the saint's reply. He had no further questions for the saint, but he continued the discussion for the pure joy of hearing the saint's remarks.

"A king has vast wealth," the king said. "You're an emperor. You must have more wealth than a king."

"I do," the saint said. "A king is a prisoner. Thus, he's unhappy. Only one who is unhappy accumulates wealth. Only one who has expenses needs wealth. I don't have any expenses, so I don't need any money. I don't hoard or store anything, either. An emperor is someone who has no possessions and is unattached to possessions. No one in the world is wealthier than he is."

The king enjoyed this satsang very much.

"Surely, you must have a large kingdom," he said with a laugh, "And if so, naturally you must have a large army."

"Army?" The saint retorted with a frown. "Who needs an army? Only a person with enemies needs an army. I don't have any enemies. Why should I need an army?"

The king was overjoyed. He bowed in respect to the saint.

"Keep your bows," the saint said. "They're useless to me."

The king left feeling pleased and happy. He had received much food for thought. The saint closed his eyes and resumed his meditation while sitting on top of the dirt pile.

How can a king impress someone who wants nothing? This degree of nonattachment belongs only to great saints. We have accumulated so much. We have a list of countless attachments in our memory from countless lifetimes. We must progress gradually from attachment to nonattachment, as much as we are able.

STORY #55

Anything we give our parents can't be considered charity. We're obliged to them for their boundless dedication to us, and anything we offer them can only be considered a credit against our debt. Not even the most powerful son could ever repay his vast debt to his parents.

MOMMY'S INVOICE

K ILLOL WAS A BRIGHT alert third grade boy. One day his math teacher taught the class how to tabulate an invoice. The teacher illustrated the lesson with the example of a businessman who had sent an employee out of town on a business trip. When the employee returned, the boss had asked the employee for an invoice of his travel expenses. The employee had written:

Travel invoice

Item	Rupees	Annas	Paise
round trip fare	5	0	0
horse coach fare	0	8	8
2 meals at hotel	3	0	0
Total	8	8	8

Signed: Hemant Joshi

The teacher gave three or four other examples of invoices, and then instructed the students to create an invoice of their own for a homework project. Killol was fascinated with this subject and prepared several invoices for homework.

Then he got the bright idea of giving his mother an invoice, too! This idea pleased him to no end. So that night he prepared an invoice for his mother and placed it on her dresser.

The next morning his mother spotted the invoice. She smiled when she saw the following bill for Killol's services:

Mommy's Invoice

Item	Rupees	Annas	Paise
1 lb eggplant	0	2	0
1 lb potatoes	0	3	0
coriander leaves	0	0	6
mint leaves	0	0	6
green peppers	0	0	6
toothpicks	0	1	0
vegetable delivery	0	1	0
laundry delivery	0	1	6
tailor delivery	0	0	6
Total	0	7	30

Signed: Killol Upadhyaya

A day passed. When Killol got out of bed the next morning, he found another invoice. This invoice was from his mother and it was for her services to Killol:

Killol's Invoice

Item	Rupees	Annas	Paise
womb storage: 9 months	0	0	0
nursing: 18 months 5 x day	0	0	0
cradle rocking: 18 months	0	0	0
diaper changing: 18 months leaves	0	0	0
feeding: 10 years	0	0	0
bathing: 10 years	0	0	0
clothing: 10 years	0	0	0
education: 10 years	0	0	6
Total	0	0	0

Signed: Sudhabahen Upadhyaya

The moment Killol read the invoice he felt faint with remorse. Picking up the invoice, he ran into his mother's room and burst into tears.

"Mommy! Mommy!"

She kissed him all over his cheeks and burst out crying, too.

"Mommy," he said, between sobs, "Even after doing so much for me you didn't charge me for anything on your whole invoice."

"My son," she said, kissing him over and over, "I don't want any rupees, or annas, or anything else. All I want is Killol."

Overjoyed, Killol replied,

"Mommy, I don't want anything for what I do either. All I need is Mommy."

Mother and son hugged each other tightly and were deep in the ocean of love.

STORY #56

In ancient India many kings were initiated into religious life at age 51, when they retired. They walked into the forest lived in a simple dwelling and pursued the sadhana of liberation. Numerous Brahma Rishis enlightened with the Supreme Spirit also inhabited the forests. They were personifications of Brahma and were lights of knowledge, yoga, devotion, dedication, and nonattachment. Although these sages had powerful emperors as disciples, they observed the vow of renunciation and asceticism and wore only a loincloth. True asceticism differs from willful sacrifice. Asceticism is a state wherein desire for worldly pleasures, whether they are available or not, doesn't arise at all. Asceticism is a synonym for renunciation. As our love for God increases, attraction for worldly pleasures is destroyed. Asceticism means the actual dislike of worldly pleasures and extreme liking for God.

KING SHIVAJI AND THE SAINT

ONCE UPON A TIME during the medieval period of India, there lived a famous king named Chatrapati Shiva who founded the state of Maharashtra. His guru was Puissant Ramdas, a famous, but discreet, nonattached saint. Traditionally such nonattached saints lived unencumbered by worldly luxuries. Even though they had wealthy land-owning disciples, they subsisted on alms.

One day at noon King Shiva was riding from the forest toward his palace. He happened to see his guru, Ramdas, standing at the doorway of an ordinary house waiting for alms. King Shiva stopped, bowed down with devotion, and then wondered,

"Why should my gurudev bear the pain of the scorching summer heat to solicit alms? After all, I could always just send alms to his residence."

King Shiva, however, didn't want to disturb his guru by talking. So he continued riding toward the palace without saying anything to Ramdas. From then on, however, the King arranged his schedule so he could catch a glimpse of his guru at noon each day. He continued this for six months.

One day King Shivaji's heart jumped for joy. His guru was approaching the palace from a distance. Guru Ramdasji sometimes begged for alms at the palace in the same manner in which he approached any other place. As usual, he waited in the courtyard chanting the name of God. King Shivaji and his mother, Queen Dowager, approached Ramdasji a few moments later with a plate of food. The Queen put the alms into the guru's begging bowl and as she did, the King quickly pressed a letter into gurudev's hand.

"Son," Guru Ramdasji said, handing the letter back to the king, "Please read what is written in the letter."

At first, the King hesitated, but then he proceeded to read. The letter revealed that along with the alms, the King had offered his entire kingdom to his guru.

Laughing soundly, guru Ramdasji asked,

"And now what will you do?"

"I'll serve at your holy feet," replied the King humbly, somewhat perplexed by the saint's response.

"Then has your kingdom become my kingdom?" Ramdasji asked affectionately.

"Yes," replied the King.

"Do you think I'll be able to rule the state?"

"Gurudev, you're all powerful!"

"But how can I rule a kingdom and lead a renunciant's life at the same time?"

"You're more intelligent than I," replied the King with assurance, "I'm sure you can do it."

"Well then, I order you to rule the state on my behalf in the same way you have been ruling."

Bowing low and touching the holy feet of his guru, the King murmured reverently,

"As you order."

Guru Ramdasji returned to his hut.

The next day, Shivaji hoisted a saffron-colored flag and proclaimed across the land:

"Henceforth, I do not own this kingdom. It belongs to Revered Gurudev. I'm his disciple and servant."

There's a deeper meaning to this story. We should first try to master our duties or calling in life, that is, become a king of our own world, before we attempt heavy sadhana , that is, retire to the forest. The ego-purification and profound lessons learned, such as patience, endurance, tolerance, will power, selfless service, joy, prayer, nonattachment, unshakable yamas and niyamas, and lack of greed, anger, and lust build a vessel capable of God Consciousness.

STORY #57

A one-rupee note, a five-rupee note, a ten-rupee note, a fifty-rupee note, a hundred rupee-note, a thousand-rupee note, are all called notes. But they don't have the same value. Similarly, everyone's compassion is called compassion, but they don't have the same value. The compassion of a mighty person is like a valuable currency note from which a suffering person receives much benefit.

THE MIGHTY KING SAVES A BOY

ONCE UPON A TIME a King was having a new palace built on a section of his estate. Whenever he found time he would walk alone to the site and check on the progress of his new palace.

One day while inspecting the site, the King heard a child crying.

The foundation of the palace had a basement. The staircase down to the basement wasn't finished yet, so the masons used a ladder which they removed at the end of each day.

The eight year-old son of a carpenter had been playing at the site and had fallen asleep in the basement. When it was time to go home, his father didn't see his son and had assumed the boy had already gone home.

When the boy awoke, he found no one around and no way to climb out; so he cried for help in a pathetic voice.

The King heard him. The heartrending cries of the child melted his heart. Guessing that this was a workman's son, the King decided to rescue the boy, himself, rather than wait for one of his subordinates and order him to do the task.

The King approached the boy, knelt down in the dust and extended his own hand. The child grasped the King's hand and the King lifted the boy out of the basement.

Just then the King's chief minister arrived and witnessed the scene. The minister was touched by the King's empathy.

"Your Excellency!" He said. "You're so compassionate and this child is so fortunate! You have voluntarily extended your hand of royal support to this fortunate child. This is the same hand, the same royal support, that thousands of people every day are striving to obtain."

In Indian marriage ceremonies the bridegroom accepts the hand of the bride. The bridegroom's gesture symbolizes his deepest feelings and acceptance of his bride's heart, love, and life. When the Lord, Guru, or King accepts someone's hand, it's similarly symbolic. In such instances, they shower grace or bestow blessings on the person.

"Find this child's father," the King said. "Have the state arrange to pay for his studies, marriage, living expenses, and every other possible need."

Thus an ordinary event turned into an extraordinary occasion.

STORY #58

THE BLESSINGS OF MY FATHER

I WAS ONLY SEVEN years old when my father passed away, so I never had the opportunity to serve him. Due to his generous nature, he was heavily in debt upon his death. This caused him grief for he was concerned about what would happen to his children after his death.

Finding himself in such depressing situation, he had nothing to give us except his blessings. It was because of these blessings that my brother and I were able to become saints.

Well-wishing and a blessing may appear to be the same, but they aren't. Well-wishing comes from the surface of the mind, but a blessing comes from the depth of the heart. Well-wishing is like a bubble. A blessing is like a pearl. A stone can be thrown in many ways, weakly with our bare hand, or powerfully with a slingshot or a catapult. The momentum of each varies as the stone travels. Good wishes are like stones thrown by a weak arm, but blessings are like stones shot from a catapult. Those potent blessings generate faith and determination in the recipient and are never given in vain.

When I was young, I used to think if only my father had been rich, I would have been able to get a formal education and would have developed aptitudes and interests in various areas. I wasn't able, then, to appreciate my devout father. When I began to practice yoga sadhana after initiation into sanyas, however, I realized that my devout father had bestowed immeasurable spiritual wealth upon me, that he had truly blessed me.

Even after coming to a prosperous country like America, I haven't had a desire to go anywhere or see anything. Nor am I attracted to anything. I'm interested only in my sadhana. I consider this to be the miracle of my father's blessings.

Although I was only seven years old at the time, I remember all the details of his passing. My mother, father, and I were the only ones in the house. My acutely ill father was sleeping on a mat on the floor. Close to where he was sleeping there was a door which adjoined a middle room. My dejected mother was sitting in the doorway.

I was dear to my father, so I was sitting close to him. He realized that he would live only a few more days, so he constantly caressed my hand affectionately. Due to my love for him, I would sleep beside him and embrace him.

He was in intense physical pain and it was difficult for him to speak. He vacillated between consciousness and semi-consciousness. Whenever he came to his senses, his mental pain increased. My mother and I attended to him constantly. All of a sudden he opened his eyes, became alert, and saw my mother sitting in the doorway. He continued to gaze at her for a while and then tears began to flow from his eyes. My mother and I broke into tears, as well. My mother wiped away his tears with her sari.

Father spoke in a choked voice.

"I'm without wealth, so I can't leave anything behind for you. And since there are a lot of debts, you'll suffer more. I'm helpless. I'm not able to do anything at all. Nevertheless, the God to whom I've prayed day after day throughout my life is omnipotent. He'll protect you."

Then looking at me, he said to my mother,

"I think this child will bring good fortune to our family."

I sincerely believe that with those words, he conveyed all his blessings. It's for this reason that I'm sitting on a high seat in front of you. If you want to worship Truth, begin with the sacred commandment:

"Know your parents as gods."

STORY #59

I was raised with so much love. Even now when I think of it, my
eyes fill with tears. I had one brother. He was older than me. He
had a saintly character and was also an excellent musician and
poet. This is a story about a disagreement I had with him once.
We never fought over money or land or material possessions.
Whatever was mine, was his, and he felt the same way about me.
But sometimes we differed over spiritual principles.

MY BROTHER AND HIS CIGARETTES

W HEN I BECAME A swami my brother left home, too.
After being so close growing up, we saw little of each
other, then.

But I saw him once in the town of Vamli. He worshiped Lord
Vishnu and I noticed that he had a bundle of Indian cigarettes on
his altar.

"Why do you put cigarettes in front of God?" I asked.

"He's not helping me break the habit," he said. "And I can't
break it by myself. So I'm offering the cigarettes to God and
then I accept them back as His gift to me, and then I continue
smoking."

"Don't you feel that this is breaking the rule of the Shastras?"
I asked.

"I don't care at all about the written Shastras anymore!" He
said with great anger. "I believe in the religion of love! I do what
my heart says, that's all!"

"Do you believe the inner voice is always pure?" I asked. "Can
you always believe it?"

He got even more angry.

"Your God may not smoke, but my God smokes! He also
smokes hashish! And also drinks! Your God may become impure
by these things, but my God doesn't! He's the God incarnate of
purity! He purifies everyone and isn't polluted by anything!"

"Brother!" I said, and I was angry now, too, "The religion of love didn't start with you! Thousands of people have followed the path of love before you were born! I'm younger than you, but I've studied the Shastras with great faith. Someone who offers the smoke of a cigarette instead of the smoke of incense to God isn't a devotee; he's an addict! By offering the cigarettes to God you're admitting defeat to your mind. One who's a slave to his mind can never become a true devotee of God!"

My older brother didn't say anything. I picked up my few things and walked away. I left town still feeling that he was insulting and weak minded.

One year went by.

Then by chance we met in Dakol. He held my feet together and cried.

"Excuse me for that day," he said.

"Excuse me, too," I said, and we both cried openly and forgave each other.

STORY #60

*Once somebody asked my Dadaguruji: "Why do you like Swami
so much? Why do you favor him? Does he have something special
about him?" "He dwells very intently on the important matters,"
Dadaguruji replied. "He tries hard to understand the deep meaning of things and he doesn't adopt anything without understanding
the deeper meaning of it. After understanding the value of it, he
doesn't give it up even in the face of death. This is his specialness."*

*Although at first I couldn't accept this opinion of me, now after
many years of yoga sadhana I believe that this is a special quality
of my nature. The follower of this path must have this quality.
You must do yoga sadhana patiently with proper understanding.*

THE BOY WHO SOILED HIS PANTS

ONCE WHEN I WAS a young swami, I was visiting the town
of Sisogra. There was a 14 year old boy there who liked
to be at my side. That particular year there was a poor
mango crop, so the people of the town used to ration their mangoes
and bring some to me. I used to give some of the mangoes to this
boy.

I stayed for about 14 or 15 days. Then I left for a neighboring
town about 5 miles away.

"Bapuji," this boy said as I was leaving, "I would like to come
with you so that I can keep eating mangoes."

"That's fine," I said. "You can come."

The neighboring town wasn't far away and we arrived there
shortly. The people there had arranged for me to lead spiritual
discussions and I told the organizers,

"Please, if you can, give mango juice to this boy twice a day, in
the morning and in the evening. He loves mangoes."

"Yes, Bapuji," they said. "We'll do that."

They gave the young boy a room in the ashram where I was staying and he received mango juice twice a day, morning and evening. He was happy.

One day, the ashram workers were cleaning all the bathrooms and all the water pots that are used in bathrooms in India. Suddenly this boy called to me.

"Bapuji!" He called. "I have to go to the bathroom real bad! I can't hold it any longer! What should I do?"

"Here!" I said quickly, "Take this big water pot with you and go outside. There's a bathroom there."

"No!" He said, "That pot's too big! I'll spill all the water!"

"Then just run outside quickly and I'll follow with the pot," I said.

My room was on top of a hill near the temple of Madhu and you had to go down a few steps to get outside. Mango juice is purgative and the boy lost control going down the steps and soiled his pants. He turned to me full of rage.

"Why did you tell these people to bring me so much mango juice? They force me to drink it twice a day!"

"No," I said softly. "It's you who doesn't know how to drink the juice."

This same thing will happen in yoga sadhana. Everything must be done with proper understanding and great patience.

STORY #61

Soil gives life to a tree and the tree continues to live as long as it receives nourishment from the soil. Our soul gives life to our mind and our mind will live elevated and purified only to the extent that it inclines towards our soul. To elevate and purify our mind we should contemplate scriptures, repeat japa, pray, and keep good company. These practices will eliminate the dreadful shadow of sorrow.

A MOTHER CONVERTS HER WAYWARD SON

NILAMBA WAS THE ONLY beloved son of a widowed mother. He was also strong willed and disobedient. He wandered about in his youth and didn't complete his studies. He joined a group of rough young men, people with bad characters. He gambled, drank, stole, and fought. These were his favorite activities.

His mother's name was Haripriya. She was extremely unhappy with the bad karmas of her son. Again and again she spoke to him with great love,

"My son, you were born into a high family. Your father was a respected citizen of our city. Your actions are dishonoring his name. Please stop."

Each time her son responded with anger when he heard these words.

"Stop talking to me! You're talking too much! Keep your thoughts to yourself!"

Haripriya was devastated by her son's uncontrollable behavior, but she kept silent. She finally resorted to quiet prayer in front of her favorite deity. Often she sobbed.

One day, Nilamba was having a secret conversation with his rough friends. Haripriya was in the next room and she knew the group was up to no good. She hid herself close to the wall where she could hear their conversation and she was stunned to hear her son say that he was going to kill a man. He had made a bet with his friends. Haripriya had never dreamed, not in her wildest imagination, that her son had sunk to such a level of violence.

Night came. Haripriya couldn't sleep. At midnight Nilamba came out of his room ready to kill a man. It was pitch black. Nilamba opened his bedroom door quietly, certain that his mother asleep.

But Haripriya was sitting by the front door wide-awake. She had lit a small lamp in the house and Nilamba saw his mother in the light next to the door.

"My son," Haripriya begged, grabbing Nilamba's feet. "I know what you're going to do. Please stop; don't do this thing. No one is dearer to me than you. I have little regard for my life other than to love you and keep you from harm. I'm begging you. Stay home tonight. Don't go out and carry out your plans."

Haripriya's words pierced the heart of her young, violent son, but his promise to his friends won out and he roughly pushed aside his elderly mother, first lightly and then with all his strength to free his feet from her grasp.

Haripriya fell back and struck her head with great force against their stone steps. Nilamba stepped over her with no regard whatsoever for her condition, but then he too tripped and fell.

"My son," Haripriya called in the darkness with great tenderness. "Are you hurt?"

Nilamba got up and then he saw the blood streaming down his mother's face. Her eyes were full of tenderness for him and in that moment his heart opened and arrogance left him, defeated by love. He bent down and embraced his mother and wept for his wasted life and his heart was transformed.

He carried his mother inside and there she died from the blow to her head. Nilamba wept bitterly, his heart shattered to pieces. He gazed at his mother's face and bowed down to her.

"Mother," he whispered. "I've given you nothing but pain and suffering my whole life, but now I repent. I'll give peace to your soul. I'll make my character pure. I'll become a saint. I'll always remember I'm the son of a Divine Goddess."

And that is what he did.

The seeker who serves his mother and attains her blessings is truly a man of good fortune.

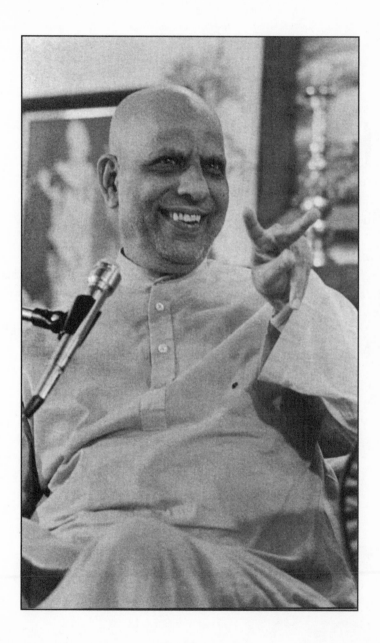

STORY #62

A NEW YEAR'S BLESSING

December 23rd, 1979

THE NEW YEAR IS coming closer with a slow step. It's coming slowly, so you can make yourself new. The Indian new year is a social celebration, but your new year is a religious celebration because it includes the birth of a great Master.

Holy Christ, the incarnation of love, gave two basic principles to the world: love and service. Love is God, and Service is our puja, or worship to Him. All other principles are included in these two.

You need not find love outside yourself. That love is already hidden in your heart. You have to awaken it and radiate its light outward.

May the New Year bring you happiness.

May your humanitarian qualities increase.

May the flower of your love bloom and may its fragrance spread everywhere.

This is my blessing and good wishes to you.

Your Beloved Grandfather,

Jai Bhagwan.

STORY #63

*Both suffering and happiness are necessary for personal growth.
Happiness comes at the end of suffering and suffering comes at the
end of happiness. No one suffers either pain or enjoys happiness
forever. Liberation means the total eradication of suffering. It's
attained only through discriminate knowledge. Only a rare yogi
receives such perfect knowledge, but every human being invariably
is blessed with a divine ray of knowledge at some point in their
life. This knowledge doesn't come from books, but from a genuine
experience and it doesn't lose its effects for as long as we live.*

THESE DAYS WILL ALSO PASS AWAY

KRISHNAKANT WAS THE SON of an aristocrat. Three years
ago his father died and with him the family fortune also
died, as his father suffered critical business losses shortly
before his death.

Krishnakant was in his last year of college at the time. He was
an honest, loving young man and he decided to repay all of his
father's debts by selling the family property. He did that and the
family was free of debt, but now they all lived in a tiny house---
Krishnakant, his widowed mother, and his younger sister.

When his family was wealthy, many aristocrats were eager to
marry their daughters to Krishnakant; but now when his wealth
was gone, their eagerness completely vanished, too. In addition,
even though Krishnakant's younger sister was well-educated, the
family poverty made marriage for her a problem, too.

These were the circumstances that lead Krishnakant to experience shame and dishonor. Even though the poverty was imposed
on him by events beyond his control, he couldn't cope with the
situation and reacted with pain and shame.

One day, because of his prior wealthy status, Krishnakant was
invited to a meeting convened by the highest dignitaries of the

city. Part of him was afraid to attend because now he was poor, and yet to decline such an invitation would have been improper.

So Krishnakant attended, but he sat nervously at the edge of the assembly not wanting any attention on himself. The hall was luxurious with a thick carpet and beautiful chandeliers and meant only for the rich and he felt out of place.

The purpose of the meeting was to establish a new college in their town. The organizers of the event had a list of the richest people in town and had invited them for the purpose of seeking donations for the new school.

When the meeting began, the secretary stood up and read each name on the list. Then he wrote down the amount of the pledge. Krishnakant listened politely and then to his horror, he heard,

"Shrikant!" This was his father's name and because of his father's worthiness and revered status, his name was still on the list of important people.

Krishnakant froze. Then with apprehension he rose from his seat.

"I pledge 1,000 rupees," he said, trying to keep his voice strong. "And I'lll pay that amount within one month."

One of Krishnakant's collegemates was also attending the assembly. His name was Manmathkumar. He had become rich, not by the strength of his character, but only after his father had died. The boys hadn't been friends in school. Krishnakant had far more talent, in art, public speaking, writing, sports, and a far superior character, even though Krishnakant had remained humble.

Manmathkumar had always been jealous. So now his face twisted into an ugly frown.

"How can this beggar donate 1,000 rupees?" He shouted. "On the contrary, we should donate something to his begging bowl!"

The entire assembly was stunned. They knew the truth about Manmathkumar and his money. His father had declared bankruptcy and had run from his debts and cheated dozens of creditors out of money he owed to them, while Krishnakant had repaid every cent of his father's debts by voluntarily accepting poverty.

"Manmathkumar!" Someone finally said. "It isn't right to say such bitter words. The ups and downs of fortune come into everyone's life. No one has ever permanently owned Laxmi, the Goddess of Fortune, nor will anyone ever own her. It isn't wise to be conceited because of your money."

The meeting ended and Krishnakant headed home devastated and humiliated. Furthermore, he had no idea where he would get 1,000 rupees within a month. Even 25 rupees would be unthinkable for his family, let alone a thousand. They were that poor.

So walking home that night, Krishnakant totally gave up. He lost hope. He couldn't stand the shame and dishonor anymore. He hated his wretched life and everything that had happened to him. He couldn't swallow the bitter pill of poverty and family dishonor anymore.

He tried to sleep that night, but couldn't. Early the next morning, tired and dejected, he awoke. It was four a.m. and he went to the river to bathe. Then he entered a nearby temple and decided to hang himself.

He had a strong rope and began his final prayers. It was still dark and a ghee lamp was lit in the temple. As he ended his prayers, his eyes fell on the wall of the temple. Someone had taken a piece of charcoal and had written:

"These days will also pass away."

His eyes were frozen on the words. He didn't even blink, not for many moments, but just kept staring at the words.

"These days will also pass away."

Was this a divine coincidence?

Yes, this was a message from the divine because his disturbed mind dropped his suicide plan. Krishnakant felt that this sentence had been written there for him. The sentence had nourished divine strength within him and had completely calmed his agitated mind.

"My Lord!" He prayed, falling to his knees. "I came here to end my life. Now I want to live and I'll return with a calm mind once again. I now understand what it means to dedicate one's whole life to You. Life becomes sacred, not by sacrificing my body to You in suicide, but by dedicating my whole mind to You."

Krishnakant went home at peace with his life.

Three days later a car approached his small house. Krishnakant was home. He watched his father's closest friend, Padmanabha, get out of the car. Padmanabha had lived abroad for many years and now was returning home for a visit.

Krishankant ran outside and both men embraced each other. They shared tears of joy at seeing each other. They went into the house and had a long conversation with Krishnakant's mother and sister.

"Krishnakant, my son," Padmanabha said. "I can't pass my remaining days here in the motherland. My daughter is my only child and I will feel secure by marrying her only to you. Your mother and father and I agreed upon this marriage many years ago, and they had granted permission. You and Daksha used to play together as children and she hasn't forgotten you to this very day. I was late in learning of your father's business losses and his passing away. When I received the news, I was so involved in my work abroad that I couldn't get away, no matter how much I tried. This was the only reason why I couldn't fulfill my obligation as a dear friend of your family. After I arrived here and heard the news of your critical financial situation, I felt great grief. By then I had already dedicated my estate worth billions of rupees to you, it's yours. I feel sorry that despite this wealth you had to go through such a financial crisis. But now the dark night has passed away and the bright morning is dawning."

Krishnakant's mind flashed back to the scene inside the temple. He saw Lord Shiva's statue, the temple walls, and the sentence written in charcoal illuminated by the flickering light of the ghee lamp.

"These days will also pass away."

And he was at peace with his life and lived a good life and never forgot the Lord.

STORY #64

THE DISCIPLE WHO ALMOST DROWN

THERE ONCE WAS A man who was looking for a guru. He was a serious devotee, but he had not found a guru to his liking yet. He had visited many saints in India, but he had always left unsatisfied.

His question to each saint was the same.

"How can I create a burning desire for God, one that will bring immediate results?"

No saint he visited could answer this question to his satisfaction.

One day, by chance, Ramakrishna Paramahansa, the Guru of Swami Vivekenanda was near by. This devotee asked around and found Ramakrishna. He was walking next to a river.

"Kind, sir," the devotee asked sincerely, "How can I create a burning desire for God, one that will bring immediate results?"

"Son," Ramakrishna replied sweetly. "I can't give you that answer here on the bank of the river. But come with me into the water, and I can give it to you there."

"I will do that," the devotee replied. "I'll go with you."

Ramakrishna took the man's hand and gently led him into the river. Deeper and deeper they went. Then suddenly with great force, Ramakrishna pushed the man's head under the water and held it there and wouldn't let him up! The man struggled and kicked and drank water trying to breath. Finally, just before the man drown, Ramakrishna grabbed the man by his hair and pulled him up.

"Save me! Save me!" The man screamed. "I'm drowning!"

"That's a burning desire," Ramakrishna said sweetly. "We have to cry to God from deep pain, then God will save us."

STORY #65

There's no action without reaction, no effect without a cause. This is a principle of science. God is the cause and the whole universe is the effect. Do you really think that the flower or leaf or branch is self-sustaining? No, the roots sustain them. In the same way our root is Almighty God and He sustains us. One of the highest principles of bhakti is: The Almighty Lord is protecting the entire universe. Try not to worry so much. Have faith in God and continue to do your work.

THE SAINT AND THE BUNDLE OF GRAIN

IN A SMALL TOWN there lived an old loving saint. He made his home in the village temple. He preferred to beg for food in other towns not where he lived. So each day he would leave town and then return home after receiving food.

Each day he received what he needed. But one day he was given a special package, a bundle full of grain. The old saint carried this bundle with him on the horse that he rode from town to town. As he traveled back toward his home, he began thinking about the grain.

"How selfish I am!" He said. "How cruel! The horse I'm sitting on is pregnant. It isn't right for me to sit on her and also carry this extra weight. She's carrying enough weight as it is."

So in order to remove the burden from his horse, he put the bundle on his own head.

He continued traveling toward home, sitting on his horse with the package of grain on his own head. Soon he met a devotee who looked upon this scene and couldn't understand what the saint was doing. When the saint approached him, the devotee asked,

"Guruji, why are you carrying that bundle on your head?"

"My mare is pregnant," the saint said. "If I allow her to carry the bundle, the load will be too much for her."

"But Guruji," the devotee answered, "You and the bundle are both on the mare!"

Sometimes we're all like this saint. If God is taking care of us, why should we worry and carry our burdens on our own head? Try not to unnecessarily worry about anything. Is there a need for a lamp to see the sun? No. When we worry about anything, it's the same thing as a crazy man trying to see the sun with the help of a lamp.

Story #66

*Pride blocks the path of knowledge. A humble individual is greatly
loved by God and the universe. Pride is the unpenetrable layer of
ignorance. Where there's no humility, spiritual knowledge doesn't
find a home. If the full cup of milk is on top and the empty bowl
is on the bottom, the milk will flow from the cup into the bowl. If
the empty cup is on top and the bottom bowl is full, the empty cup
remains empty. In the same manner, an egotistical disciple doesn't
receive knowledge from his Guru.*

The Proud District Governor

ONCE A WELL-KNOWN SAINT arrived in a big city in India.
The news of his coming spread throughout the town and
hundreds of people came for his darshan. Someone told
the District Governor.

"Sir, you should know that an important saint has arrived in
our city."

The District Governor nodded in affirmation. After asking
several questions about the saint, he decided it would be worthwhile to visit him.

This was the during the time when India was ruled by the
British government. This particular District Governor was an
Indian, appointed by the British to head this district. It was his
duty to administer justice and to collect taxes for the British government. During this time, there were few Indians who had studied English, so anyone with a working knowledge of the language
could get a job immediately. Under those circumstances, of course,
Indians who had studied English were proud of themselves. As
you might imagine, if these workers rose to a high office, their
pride rose with them.

Thus, this District Governor was very proud. Summoning
one of his rich friends, he asked,

"Do you usually go for the darshan of that famous saint who is visiting our city?"

"Yes, sir, I do. Would you like to go with me?"

"Yes, but I'll go on my own terms. I can't go among a mass of people and just sit anywhere. I must go within the proper protocol."

"Rest assured," his friend said, "I'll make all the appropriate arrangements for your arrival by contacting the organizers and the city officials. When do you plan to go?"

"I'll arrive on Sunday at 6 p.m. By that time the saint will be through with his discourse, and most of the people will have gone home. It's all right if twenty-five to fifty people remain, but I wish to have a personal conversation with the saint."

"I'll arrange it for you," his friend said.

That Sunday, the District Governor left for darshan at the appointed time. When the saint's discourse ended, the assembly dispersed with the exception of about fifty close disciples who sat close to the saint. When the District Governor's car arrived, about a dozen gentlemen disciples came to greet him. They courteously escorted him into the presence of the saint.

The District Governor bowed down to the saint and sat close to him. After a few moments he said to the saint,

"I've had a strong desire to visit you, but my busy schedule has prevented me from doing so. During your public talks, you probably give common teachings, so how would I benefit by visiting you anyway during those times? Thus, I decided to visit Your Excellency in relative privacy. By the way, I've read many scriptures related to knowledge, devotion, and yoga. These contain all there is to know. I've come to you, however, looking for inspiration. Please grace me by teaching me what I personally need to know."

The saint listening silently.

Just as the ocean is fed by many streams and yet is one, so a saint is fed by the experiences of many people and yet is just one person. In other words, a great saint is an ocean of human experience. Thus, he easily detected that the District Governor was filled with pride.

What can you put into a full pot? It must be emptied first before it can be filled. This the great saint knew.

"Practice saying Ram, Ram," the saint said lovingly.

The District Governor burst into laughter. In his opinion, only common people chanted the Lord's name. Intellectual people needed an advanced technique.

"I already know that!" He replied pertly. "So what else is new? Tell me something that's appropriate for my stage."

The saint remained serene. Then suddenly he said forcefully, "Fool!"

Everyone was shocked! The saint had always exhibited restraint and good manners. He had never ridiculed even a common person before, not even in private, and yet today he had publicly insulted a government official!

The District Governor fumed at the insult. It was intolerable to him that a person of his status should be publicly ridiculed by someone wearing a mere loincloth. His ego, intoxicated by a sense of superiority, became inflamed and his facade of good manners totally collapsed.

"Are you insulting me?" He shouted, and his body trembled violently. "Who are you to insult me? How could a so-called saint act like this?"

"I haven't insulted anyone," the saint said calmly. There wasn't the slightest hint of any fight or argument in the saint's voice.

"What!" The District Governor shouted, "You haven't insulted me?"

"No, I haven't insulted you," the saint replied.

"You're Lying!"

"I don't lie."

"Didn't you just call me a fool?"

"I definitely used the word fool," the saint replied serenely. "You certainly know the word fool. As soon as I said the word your face got red, your body trembled with anger, and your mind became enraged. Yes, it seems that you're well acquainted with the word fool. But brother, you told me that you know the word Ram. I don't think you know the word Ram at all. If you really did know Ram, your eyes, your body, and your heart would have responded much differently. You would have remained calm. So, dear brother, you should repeat Ram, Ram, Ram. Repeating the sound Ram is the first step in spiritual sadhana. Right now you're a beginner on the spiritual path. If you had been a sadhak of high standard, the word Ram would have protected your mental state."

After hearing the sweet speech of the saint, the District Governor's anger subsided. He realized his mistake and everyone realized that the saint hadn't expressed genuine dislike or anger, but had pretended to do so to induce anger in the District Governor. Without such dramatics, it would have been impossible to answer the District Governor's question.

We all go through such dramas, whether we want to or not. Sometimes our dramas are clearly a melodrama to us and don't fool us or disturb our minds. At other times our dramas appear real and disturb us very much. In those moments, keep silent and remember your mantra. Just as the north star indicates the direction of true north, your mantra continually points toward your goal, peace.

STORY #67

*If we touch a shaven head in the darkness, should we believe
we've touched a saint? If we see long hair swaying on someone's
shoulders during the daylight, should we believe we've seen a saint?
How can we recognize a saint? Should we look for saffron clothes
or tilak on a person's forehead? No, a saint isn't recognized by his
body, but by his temperament. What's in the mind of ordinary
people isn't in their speech, and what's in their mind and speech
isn't in their conduct. But the thought, speech, and conduct of a
saint are harmoniously synchronized.*

THE FOUR FAKE SAINTS

ONCE THERE WERE FOUR friends who graduated from college together. They were lazy and neglected their work.
This prevented them from getting or holding jobs. When they were hired, they didn't last long because they were jealous, arrogant, and deceitful. Their behavior polluted whatever environment they worked in. Although they repeatedly lost their jobs, they didn't change their behavior. They were all intelligent, actually, but their intellect had been diverted into a wrong channel.

One day when they were traveling together they saw throngs of people headed toward a temple. They were curious, so they asked a passer-by,

"Where's everyone going?"

"To the discourse of a famous saint," came the reply.

The friends looked at each other. They were unemployed with lots of time on their hands and they were bored, as usual, so one of them said,

"Let's go hear the saint, too. It'll give us something to do."

The others agreed.

Mingling with the crowd, they eventually arrived at the temple.

The saint started his talk. He was an older, scholarly sanyasi who directed an ashram and various public activities in the area. His talk touched the hearts of everyone. The audience couldn't get enough of his sweet speech.

The four friends were influenced by the discourse, too. They watched with special interest as the audience heaped large garlands of flowers, fruit, sweets, and money at the saint's feet. Immediately they decided to become renunciates, for they thought it would be the easiest way to become rich. However, they were only after wealth and pleasure. Even if religion and liberation had been handed to them free of charge, they would have had no desire to accept them.

After the discourse the four men went into seclusion. They talked late into the night for many nights on how to become fake swamis.

Fifteen days later, the four men set forth on their journey to become sanyasis. They traveled to a place where no one knew them, 800 miles from their hometown, and started living in a deserted Shiva temple. They each put ash over their body, dressed in a loincloth and carried a begging bowl when they left the Shiva temple.

The most deceitful of the four young men became the guru. He called himself, guru Maharaj, and the other three became his disciples. While guru Maharaj remained inside the deserted Shiva temple, the other three men went their separate ways to beg alms in different sections of the city.

One day one of the men approached a house with his begging bow. He chanting the name of the Lord and then stood silently. A man and his wife, standing in their courtyard, saw the begging bowl in the sanyasi's hand and knew that he had come for alms. His manner was graceful and he appeared detached from the external world. They gave the fake swami food and then said kindly,

"Welcome, swamiji."

The fake swami stood a few moments as if in deep contemplation and then accepted their invitation and walked into their small house.

"Please be seated," the husband said, pointing to a swing reserved for guests.

The swami seated himself on the swing.

"Swamiji," the husband continued, "Where are you from?"

Noticing that the master of the house spoke Gujarati, the fake swami replied,

"I don't speak Gujarati very well, but I'll try, since that's your language. Brother, I'm a swami. I wander constantly from place to place. I don't believe in any type of bondage to this world. I stay longer in places where my yoga meditation is most successful."

The owner of the house was extremely impressed with the swami's pure pronunciation of Gujarati. Actually all four men were from the state of Gujarat.

"Your pronunciation indicates that you've studied the language. You must be a learned scholar. Although we speak Gujarati here, we ourselves can't pronounce it as precisely as you."

"This is due to the profound grace of my most reverend gurudev," the swami said in a solemn voice.

Meanwhile, the wife came out with a plate of food and the husband reverently asked,

"Swamiji, if you would grace us by eating here, we would be extremely pleased."

The swami placed his palm lovingly on the husband's shoulder and said,

"I'm not alone. I have two guru brothers and reverend gurudev with me, as well. We take alms only after offering the food to gurudev."

"Then please accept more alms," the husband insisted.

"No," the swami replied, "That isn't necessary. My guru brothers have also gone to other parts of the city today to seek alms. Gurudev is a great yogi. He'll eat a little if we really insist. The alms we bring back are usually enough for us."

With that he extended his alms bowl and accepted the food placed on it.

The husband was impressed by the swami's verbal skills. Believing the swami was a yoga sadhak and that his guru was also an accomplished yogi, the husband expressed sincere interest in yoga.

"Swamiji, I'm extremely fond of yoga. I've read many books on the subject, but since I haven't been able to find a genuine guide, I haven't been able to begin my yoga practice."

"Then come to the deserted Shiva temple after 5:00 this afternoon. Gurudev spends the whole day in yoga practice and comes out only for a short time."

"I've read yoga books only in English," the husband said.

"That's fine," the swami said. "Most Reverend Gurudev is omniscient. I believe he knows every language in the world, although he doesn't go around demonstrating this fact everywhere. Let me tell you a bit about myself. When I was only twelve years old, I fell deeply in love with my guru. One night I surrendered at his feet and renounced my home. Gurudev tried to dissuade me from doing so, but I didn't return. Two years passed and he was satisfied with my service. One day he placed his gracious hand on my head, and I received the knowledge of English, Hindi, Gujarati, and other languages, although I'd only finished three grades in school."

"You really love your gurudev, don't you," the husband said.

"Gurudev is a great, divine being," the swami replied solemnly. "Whoever develops love for him will definitely reach his goals. Gurudev isn't fond of publicity, so we don't publicize his accomplishments anywhere. Occasionally, however, feelings of love overwhelm me and words of praise accidentally slip off my tongue."

Then the fake swami left, returning that night to the deserted Shiva temple.

In just two weeks, the three disciples had transformed Guru Maharaj into an accomplished yogi by spreading various rumors. Inhabitants of the city were filled with devotion. Throngs of people began to come for the darshan of guru Maharaj.

In addition, the three disciples began giving discourses every Sunday. One disciple gave his talks in Hindi. Another disciple gave his talks in English. The third disciple gave his talks in Gujarati."

Within six months, the four young men were the center of discussion in every home. "Guruji," a rich townsman said one day, "With the touch of your holy feet, the whole city has been transformed into the home of the Lord. I'm planning to buy land and have the necessary buildings constructed for an ashram."

"No, brother, no," Guru Maharaj said. "Don't bind a nonattached person like me to the bonds of an ashram. We swamis are like the birds of the air, here today, gone tomorrow. Because of the love of everyone here, we'll stay as long as possible, but then we'll move on. You may buy land, if you wish. Have some huts built on it, but don't plan to construct permanent dwellings."

"As you wish, gurudev," the rich man replied.

Every day fruits and sweets were piled at the feet of guru Maharaj and numerous gifts poured in, as well. In the beginning, the three disciples distributed the food, clothing, and money to the poor in the presence of everyone. Then they distributed only one third of the donations and kept the remaining portion hidden in secret storage.

The four men decided to collect 800,000 rupees to divide among themselves and then leave. They planned to return home wealthy and then to spend the rest of their lives running small shops.

After three years, there wasn't anyone within a hundred miles who hadn't heard of the four men. They were such proficient actors that everyone considered them to be simple, loving, innocent, nonattached saints who were devoted to the Lord.

But then the four swamis got tired of it all: covering their bodies with ash, wearing only loincloth, begging for food. They decided that they had enough money hidden away, so they decided to leave town the next day.

In a nearby city, however, there lived a miserly rich man who never spent money for religious purposes. He had heard that the four saints were nonattached and would either return whatever wealth they received or distribute it among the poor. He knew that a wealthy person had once donated 1,000 rupees, and another time a rich man had donated 5,000 rupees, and yet the saints had declined the donations saying each time,

"Brother, this money isn't needed now, so just keep it with you. We'll let you know if we need it."

When he heard these things, the miser had an idea.

"The people believe that I'm a miser," he said, "If I donate 10,000 rupees to that saint, he won't accept such a huge amount and I'll gain great influence in society."

So, the next day, when a large group of people had gathered to hear guru Maharaj speak, the rich miser arrived with ten porters. Each porter carried a bag of 1,000 rupees in coins on his head. The people were astonished.

"When did that old miser become so generous?" They asked.

One of the town dignitaries whispered into guru Maharaj's ear.

"This man with the bags of money? He's stingy. Don't return the money to him."

Guru Maharaj smiled, only too happy to agree with the man, knowing full well that the four fake saints were about to leave town, and now they could leave richer than ever.

"Oh, all right," Guru Maharaj whispered back. "I'll do as you wish."

The porters placed the bags of money at Guru Maharaj's feet.

"Dear disciples!" Guru Maharaj called, and the three disciples hurriedly came and bowed down to him.

"Gurudev, do you have instructions for us?" One of the disciples asked.

"Yes. This wealthy gentleman has so lovingly offered this gift that we must accept it. Please take the bags of money and bring them into the ashram."

"As you wish, Gurudev," and the disciples disappeared with the money.

Regretting his foolishness, the miser said,

"Dear Saints, I thought you were nonattached and had renounced wealth."

"Dear Tycoon," one of the disciples responded, "You should chant Ram, Ram. What do you mean we saints are nonattached? We're totally attached! Yes, we can easily renounce one, two, or three rupees. But it's a different story to renounce bags and bags of thousands of rupees. On the contrary, I would say that you're the nonattached person. Even though you're not wearing a loincloth, you seem to have no regard for money."

The miser realized he had been deceived, but he was unable to regain a single rupee. A few days later, guru Maharaj told the townspeople,

"Dear friends, I'm so weary of all this activity. I've performed as much social service as I can. Now I long to pass the rest of my life in a secret place at Uttarkashi in the Himalayas. I haven't decided when I'll leave, but when I go, don't allow any pain to enter your minds at all. We saints are like birds from the realm of the Lord, and now we're reminded of that heavenly place. Our minds have become overwhelmed, so we're not certain at what moment we'll extend our wings and fly away."

On the very next day the huts stood empty, with not a guru or disciple to be found.

A small child doesn't become elderly if he wears the clothes of his elderly grandfather, puts grandfather's spectacles on his little nose, and tries to walk and talk like him. Similarly, no person can become a saint simply by acting like a saint in external ways. We recognize the extent of his genuineness sooner or later. To do so, however, we must come in close contact with him and even then we may be unable to recognize a genuine saint if we don't know how to identify virtues.

STORY #68

HOW TULSIDAS BECAME A SAINT

ONCE IN INDIA THERE lived a famous, high saint named, Tulsidas. He wrote a beautiful explanation of the Ramayan in Hindi that's known all over India. He's also one of India's greatest poets.

He wasn't born a saint. He was born poor, a very ordinary man. He married and he loved his wife so much that it bordered on obsession. When she got up and walked into another room in their house, he did so, too. He followed her around like that, not wanting to be out of her sight. Often he just sat and gazed at her.

"Why does he act this way?" His wife used to say. She enjoyed being loved and admired, but this was too much for her and she didn't like it. It was almost like he was crazy. But she didn't say anything to him because she didn't want to cause any pain to her husband.

One day Tulsidas had to leave the house for something. His attachment to his wife was so great that he seldom, if ever, left the house without her or allowed her to leave the house without him. On this day, though, he had to leave alone.

His wife was pleased with this. She hadn't seen her mother in a long time and decided she would visit her mother as soon as her husband left. When Tulsidas left, she left, too, walking across town to visit her mother.

When Tulsidas returned, he found the house locked and knew that his wife was visiting her mother. He was tired from the day, but left immediately overwhelmed with the desire to be with his wife.

There was a river nearby and Tulsidas had to cross it to reach the house of his mother-in-law. Rather than wait for a boat, he waded into the river and walked across it so great was his pain at being separated from his wife.

It was dark when he reached his mother-in-law's house. He was wet and cold and everyone was asleep in the house. He circled the house two or three times, deciding what to do. Indian custom said that he, as a son-in-law, should enter with dignity, not wet and cold late at night.

But he wanted to see his wife's face so bad that he climbed a high plant next to the wall and got onto the lower roof of the house. Then he grabbed what appeared to be a rope and entered the small window of the room where he knew his wife would be sleeping.

Quietly he walked over to his sleeping wife. When he saw her face, the exhaustion left his body and he became calm and content. He touched her slightly and she woke up.

She was startled to see her husband gazing at her. His clothes were wet and dirty. His hair was wild and uncombed.

"What are you doing here?" She blurted out, "And why do you look like that?"

"You tied a rope for me outside your window," Tulsidas said.

"What rope?" She asked.

They both went to the window and saw a huge snake hanging next to the wall.

Then his wife, overcome with anger, confusion, and frustration at the actions of her husband, spoke to him from her heart. The words just tumbled out.

"This body of mine is made of bones and skin and flesh! Why are you so attracted to it? If you had that much love for God, you would have found Him a long time ago and been a happy man."

Her words of truth exploded into the soul of Tulsidas and a new light filled his heart. He bowed to his wife and tears streamed down his face.

"Sister," he now called her. "You've told me the truth. Give me your blessings tonight so I can leave you as my wife and seek God."

Tulsidas never went back home again. He left that night, wet clothes and all, and started his sadhana and met God. He became one with God. This saint that I'm talking about isn't an ordinary saint; he was a high saint, one of the greatest in Indian history. He lived in seclusion for 12 years, doing nothing but sadhana, and he practiced with such intensity that he reached the feet of the Lord.

Great saints have one quality: the things that worldly people strive after appear insignificant to them. We're all travelers on the same path, so we should also learn to practice with seriousness and keep our focus on our goal. To read and listen a lot, is one thing. But to practice, even a little, is the most important. The day you begin to sincerely practice, your true progress will begin.

STORY #69

This is a true story about how little hurts can grow into big hurts.
It's something that happened in my hometown.

SOMETHING SO TERRIBLE FROM SOMETHING SO SMALL

ONCE IN MY TOWN a young couple decided to get married. They loved each other very much. Palavi, the girl, went home and told her parents her intentions. Her father was a little disturbed, as the custom at the time was for children to follow the guidance of their parents, but he accepted his daughter's wish.

"Who's the young man?" The father asked.

"I'll point him out to you," Palavi said. "I'm sure you'll like my choice. His name is Panchi."

In India marriage is more than the union of two people; it's the union of two families. The two families try to come together, as well, to love and serve each other. If there's friction between the young married couple, then there's friction between the two families, as well. Thus, the parents try to give guidance before two young people get married, as they may not understand this. But Palavi's father was willing to forgo this advice, as his daughter had already made up her mind.

Palavi brought Panchi home to meet her father. They all talked and Palavi's father liked Panchi. Likewise, Panchi brought Palavi home to meet his parents and they, too, approved of the marriage.

Shortly thereafter, the two young people were married.

For six months they were happy. Then a small incident happened. Really it was nothing but a misunderstanding.

"Today, I really want to please Panchi," Palavi decided one day and she fixed her hair a special way. She dressed it up, very artistically. Now at that time in India, the women from higher-class families never did this. It was considered bad taste, like a prostitute almost. But each generation is revolutionary in their own way. They challenge the status quo and change things and this was all Palavi was doing, in her own small way, just showing her independence.

She waited with great anticipation for Panchi to come home, certain he would like her beautiful hair. But when Panchi walked through the door and saw his wife with make up and a dashing hairstyle, he got angry.

"Why have you done all these artificial things to yourself?" He asked, "Do these things look good to you?"

Palavi was crushed. But rather than explain that she did it to please him, she got angry.

"This is my hair!" She hollered, "And I'll fix it any way I want to!"

"Oh, no you won't!" Panchi hollered back. "Women in my family don't fix their hair like this! Only prostitutes do!"

"And if I fix my hair like this then suddenly I'm a prostitute in your eyes?" She hollered. "Then I'm leaving! Good-bye!"

"Good-bye!" Panchi hollered back and Palavi left their house.

One day passed. Two days passed. Three days passed. No Palavi; she had gone home to her parents.

Fifteen days passed and still they were separated, not speaking to each other.

"Where is Palavi?" Panchi's parents kept asking, until he got tired of it and moved to a nearby town and found work as a high school teacher.

Meanwhile, Palavi stayed with her parents. Her brother was also living there with his wife and one day the sister-in-law said with great love,

"Palavi, I thought for sure that I wouldn't see you for three or four years. I was certain you wanted to be left alone with your husband, you loved him so much."

Then the whole family found out what had happened, that Palavi had annoyed her husband with a new hairstyle and they hadn't been able to make up. Panchi's family found out, as well.

Three years passed. Can you imagine, three years! And still they hadn't spoken to each other. Panchi continued to teach and all his students loved him. He was gentle and bright and wherever he went, he always had students around him, laughing and asking questions, they loved him so much.

One day the students were talking among themselves.

"Isn't our teacher married?" They asked. "Surely he must be married, someone as handsome and wonderful as him! But we've never seen him with anyone. Let's visit him at home and see if he's married."

So that evening they visited Panchi and saw that he lived alone. But they noticed a picture on his altar of a beautiful woman. Underneath the picture, he had written:

"Truly I have offended you, very badly."

Many times Panchi had wanted to write a letter to Palavi and tell her that, but his pride got in the way and he would think,

"Is it necessary for me to write a letter like this? Can't she come to me on her own without a letter from me?"

And Palavi's pride was also blocking her heart.

"Shouldn't he write me a letter?" She thought, "Or visit my parents' home and ask about me?"

But then she would think,

"How silly of me. If I had just changed my hairstyle back to how he liked it that night, none of this would have happened. Why didn't I do that? I haven't behaved properly."

She had a necklace and she kept Panchi's picture inside the locket and she would look at the picture and cry.

"Where did all this anger come from? My anger. His anger. What happened? Maybe it was me. Maybe I caused all this anger."

And then she would cry some more.

Both of them passed their days like this.

Then one day one of Panchi's students visited him after school at home. When Panchi went close to his altar, the student followed and asked,

"Whose picture is this?"

"This is my wife," Panchi replied with tears in his eyes.

"Then why isn't she living here with you?"

"Because she won't come," Panchi answered.

"Maybe you're not calling her right," the student said innocently.

The next day in school, the student told the others about the situation. They found out the name of Panchi's wife and where she lived but decided it wasn't proper to visit her.

A few weeks later, Panchi got sick. He wasn't in school and the students were worried about him. A doctor came and said,

"This is serious. He may not live. Where is his family? They should all be informed."

The students sent telegrams to all the relatives, including Palavi. She was sweeping her mother's house when she heard someone call her name.

"Palavi! I have a telegram for someone named, Palavi!"

She saw the telegram was from the town where Panchi was living. She opened it and read the news about his illness.

"Come soon," the telegram said.

She quickly packed a handbag and walked to the station. Her heart was beating heavily and her eyes were full of tears.

"How can something so terrible come from something so small?" She said.

When she arrived in Panchi's town, his students were waiting for her and recognized her from her picture.

"We have a taxi for you," they said.

"How is he?"

"He's very sick, but he'll be alright once he sees you."

They brought her to Panchi's house and she served him with great love. He opened his eyes and recognized her and they both cried.

Palavi stayed by Panchi's side for seven days and nursed him back to health.

"This is a miracle!" the doctor said, when he visited again. "I didn't think he would make it."

"You don't have to come back," the students said. "He has the right medicine now."

When Panchi was well, Palavi quietly packed her bags to leave.

"Please don't go," Panchi said. "Forgive me. It was all my fault. It was your hair. You should be able to do whatever you want with your own hair."

"No, it was my fault," she said. "I shouldn't have gotten angry over something so silly."

And they made up and lived happily together again.

How painful their suffering was, for three years over something so small. If either one of them had been more forgiving of the other, three years of terrible pain would never have happened. Be patient with each other, especially with your family. Be patient and tolerant. Love one another and be kind.

STORY #70

Many mango trees in India bear fruit twelve years after planting.
If a mango tree is planted by someone who's unaware that fruition
takes twelve years, the patience he's shown for eleven years may be
lost. He may cut down the tree just before it comes to fruition.

THE SHEPHERD BOY AND THE LOTTERY TICKET

O NCE UPON A TIME in the early morning a kind shepherd
named, Bhola, was grazing his sheep on the outskirts of
a village. A friend saw him and shouted,
"Bhola!"

Bhola looked up and saw his friend, Shankara Patel.

"Wait a minute!" Shankara called. "I have something for
you."

Bhola stopped and waited.

"What is it?" Bhola asked.

"I have two lottery tickets," Shankara said. "They only cost
one rupee each. Why don't you buy one? What's a rupee? If
you don't win, you're only out a rupee. If you do win, you'll be a
100,000 rupees richer!"

"Shankara," Bhola said. "How can a shepherd like me who
chases sheep all day be destined to win the lottery? But...you're my
childhood friend, so take this rupee."

Shankara left and bought the two lottery tickets.

When he returned he gave Bhola his ticket stub and watched
as Bhola folded it up and put the stub into his shepherd's staff for
safe keeping.

The two friends parted.

Four months later, the lottery winners were announced.

Bhola won first place, 100,000 rupees. Shankara learned the
news first and hurried to the riverbank where Bhola was grazing
his sheep.

"Bhola!" He cried. "The Lord has graced you today! You won the lottery, first place, 100,000 rupees!"

Bhola danced with joy.

"100,000 rupees!" He cried, totally out of his mind with the news. "I'm so tired of grazing sheep after all these years in all kinds of weather; winter, summer, monsoons. Now I won't have to do this anymore!" And he took his staff and threw it into the river saying, "I'm done with you!"

"No!" Shankara yelled, "Bhola, what have you done? Your lottery ticket is inside your staff! Quick, jump in and get the staff! If you don't show the ticket you can't get the prize money!"

Bhola's euphoria turned to panic. He quickly removed his clothes and jumped into the river. A few minutes later he returned with his wet staff.

"Don't remove the ticket now," Shankara scolded. "Wait until your staff has dried."

The root of patience is knowledge and tolerance, while the root of impatience is mental restlessness. When we waver just at the moment of success, we're like a ship sinking just as it reaches the shore.

STORY #71

If you find a person who arouses good feelings in you, you should regard him as your Sadguru and serve him. You must keep your-self in eternal contact with his pure soul. In the Bhagavad Gita Shri Krishna taught his dear disciple, Arjuna, how to obtain spiritual knowledge: "Dear Arjuna, go to a knowledgeable and master Guru, and receive the highest knowledge that will liberate you from suffering, by bowing down, serving him, and asking questions with humility." If a disciple doesn't love his Guru with a pure heart, he can't progress spiritually. Without love for your Guru, knowledge isn't possible. There's a great difference between conditional service and selfless service. The disciple serving selflessly is close to his Guru and he gets much greater reward than the one who serves with selfish motives.

THE DULL DISCIPLE

IN INDIA THERE LIVED a great master named Shankaracharya. He defeated all the scholars and philosophers of his day who challenged him and established his path firmly on non-duality, the belief in one God. He had a large following of disciples and taught scriptures to them.

In his group of renunciates there was a dull disciple. This particular disciple, however, had limitless faith in his Guru. He served his Guru with constant awareness and love. When the other disciples were busy with philosophical discussions, he would clean his Guru's house, wash his clothes, and keep busy with other services. He was slow mentally, though, and the other disciples laughed at his dullness.

Before each teaching session, Guru Shankaracharya liked to look around to see which disciples were present. He would always wait for the dull disciple, as this disciple was usually late. The other disciples didn't like this.

"Guruji," one of the other disciples said one day. He was a disciple who thought himself to be especially learned. "Why do you wait for him? He doesn't understand anything even when he's here. He's dumb."

Guru Shankaracharya would say nothing and continue to wait with great patience for the arrival of the dull disciple. The dull disciple sincerely tried to be on time. He never wanted to be late, but due to his boundless love for his Guru, he was always busy in some service to Him and he would forget about the time.

The other disciples scolded him constantly.

"Late again? Why are you late?" They would ask.

"Please forgive me," the dull disciple would answer, never hating the others.

One day, the dull disciple was on time. He seldom had any questions for his Guru, and seldom expressed any thought in his Guru's presence, but today, with tears in his eyes, he spoke to Guru Shankaracharya.

"Beloved Gurudev," he said. "Please forgive me. I'm dumb and don't enjoy studying the scriptures. I experience divine joy only in serving you."

Guru Shankaracharya's heart melted with love as he listening to this prayer.

"My son," he said with great tenderness. "Open your mouth."

The dull disciple opened his mouth.

The great Guru wrote the mantra, OM, on the disciple's tongue with a stick. Suddenly layers of ignorance disappeared from the disciple's mind, and the dull disciple experienced omniscience.

The next day the disciple went to the river to get some water for his Guru. The other disciples were bathing

"I hear you're the top disciple now!" They laughed. "The favorite of Guruji! If you're so smart now, why don't you chant a new song for us!"

Immediately a fountain of new chants flowed from the mouth of the dull disciple. None of the others could fathom how the dull disciple had gotten so brilliant. They were struck with awe. When they asked the disciple how he had attained his divine power, the dull disciple placed his palms together, began crying, and said in a choked voice,

"Service to the Guru."

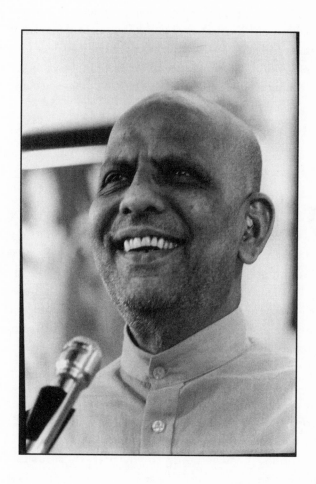

STORY #72

Silence means to control our speech. The little elf the tongue needs a giant to control it, and when the elf is angry all the ingenuity of the giant is needed to check it. God has given us a tongue so we can talk. However, it can act like a horse without a reign or a haughty elephant. Lord Krishna says in the Bhagavad Gita that if a devotee wants to feel devotion for God, he must triumph over his tongue and his genitals. Just as a dog wags his tail when he sees his owner, so our mind wags its tail at the command of these two organs.

THE BUSINESSMAN OF BENGALGRANUS AND SILENCE

ONCE UPON A TIME an orphan boy named, Mohan, lived in a city among a colony of poor people. Mohan's parents had died when he was just a little boy, and he was raised by all his neighbors who pitied him.

As Mohan grew and became a young man, he found work as a laborer. He supported himself well, and everyone loved him because he was generous, polite, tolerant, honest, and soft-spoken. Eventually he saved his wages and opened a small shop in which he sold roasted chick-peas. Mohan's honesty allowed him to rise from a laborer into a highly prosperous businessman.

After becoming prosperous, Mohan got married and eventually had three children. Every Sunday there was an open-air market in his section of the city. He would sit there with bags full of roasted chick-peas and always make a good profit.

One Sunday he was going to the market, as usual, with his cart loaded with bags of chick-peas. The market was extremely crowded that day, so to avoid an accident, he pushed his cart slowly and shouted,

"Hey, brother! Please let me by! Hey, sister! Please make way for me! Oh, mother! Please allow me to pass!"

At one intersection, the crowd was especially dense. He continued onward, still shouting, when suddenly a child ran right in front of him and was crushed to death under his cart! People gathered around screaming. The Police came.

Mohan was terribly upset. He spoke to the police and explained that it was an accident. Although he was innocent, the child's mother claimed otherwise. The two gave differing reports to the police and eventually the day was fixed for his trial.

The day before his trail, Mohan went to the Sunday market with his bags of chickpeas as usual, but his mind was worried and unsteady. Tomorrow he must stand trial. There were dark lines of grief and worry on his face and he continually prayed to God.

Then a sanyasi appeared. Many times this sanyasi had lovingly received roasted chickpeas from Mohan on a Sunday at the marketplace. The sanyasi was free of worldly desires, and Mohan and the people of the city loved him dearly. Today, like always, he lovingly accepted alms from Mohan. But then seeing Mohan's sad face, he asked,

"Brother, why are you so sad today?"

Mohan steadied his shaking voice and then told the sanyasi the entire story of his cart accident, concluding with the news that he must stand trial the next day and face the angry mother.

The sanyasi asked a few questions about the incident and then thought for a while. Finally, he asked Mohan,

"During the trial, will you behave as I advise?"

"I trust you as I do my father and mother," Mohan replied.

"Then tomorrow when the prosecuting attorney interrogates you, observe silence and continually reflect upon the Lord."

"I will follow your instructions," Mohan said humbly.

The sanyasi blessed him and then departed.

The next day Mohan went to court. First, the woman whose child had died under the cart recounted the whole incident. Her lawyer then interrogated Mohan, who remained silent and wouldn't answer a single question. Unable to tolerate Mohan's silence, the woman lost her temper. Interrupting her attorney, she loudly snapped,

"When you were on your way to the market in your cart, your voice was certainly loud enough! You could speak then! You could have broken someone's eardrum shouting, 'Make way! Make way!' Why are you playing dumb now? Why won't you speak?"

Mohan's lawyer immediately jumped to his feet,

"When Mohan was shouting so loudly for the right-of-way, while passing through the crowd, why didn't you hold your son?" He asked the woman. "Clearly you heard him shouting! Why didn't you stop your son from running so freely?"

The mother had no answer.

After hearing all the testimony, the judge declared Mohan innocent and set him free. Afterwards, Mohan's attorney asked him privately,

"Why did you observe silence?"

"A sanyasi living in our city had advised me to observe silence and reflect upon God when the prosecuting attorney interrogated me," Mohan said.

Mohan's lawyer laughed and said,

"Mohanbhai, you may not know it, but that renunciate used to be a famous trial lawyer before taking vows of sanyas. His advice clearly helped demonstrate your innocence today."

Although Mohan had observed silence for just a few moments, they were just the right moments to stay quiet. Conversely, although the irate mother had let her tongue loose for just a few moments, those were just the wrong moments to let it loose. We want peace but we aren't willing to be silent. We speak much more than necessary. Our bitter words result in quarrels. When gentle people speak it seems like a bottle of perfume has opened. But when boisterous people speak it seems like a foul-smelling sewer has opened.

STORY #73

When a highly developed yogi meditates, the yogic fire induces various types of sound to flow from his mouth. This process is called anahat nad, or spontaneous sound. All the divine mantras are manifested through anahat nad. The first syllable, usually OM, is the seed syllable. The mantra's energy resides here.
When a mantra is repeated with strong conviction , or bhavana, it strengthens our will power and purifies our mind through concentration. When a divine mantra bears fruit, the fruit is unshakable faith.

THE THREE SAINTS AND THEIR MANTRA

ONCE UPON A TIME three elderly saints lived on an isolated island. Although they were old, they lived innocent and simple lives like children, and they were frank and affectionate with everyone. Moreover, there wasn't the slightest notion in their heads that they were special in any way. Yet many people came regularly for their darshan, as their fame had spread far and wide.

One day a scholar visited the island. He hadn't come for the saints' darshan; he had come to relax and enjoy the beauty of the island. From the ship's deck, he saw the three saints and decided to remain on board to scrutinize their activities unobserved. The scholar was proud of his knowledge and considered everyone else ignorant.

Smirking to himself, he said,

"How foolish these saints are! I don't see anything special about these illiterate idiots. Yet people flock to see them. Why?"

After darshan the crowds left and the scholar sent two of his disciples to the saints.

"Today our gurudev has come to the island," the disciples told the saints. "He's a brilliant scholar and a scriptural genius."

Extremely impressed, the saints immediately left with the disciples to meet the scholar on board the ship. After bowing down to him, they sat humbly at his feet and addressed him respectfully.

"Dear scholar, you've graced us by visiting this island. We like to hear stories of the Lord. Since you're a learned scholar, please teach us some of the scriptures."

The scholar's chest puffed with pride and he taught them for a while. Eventually he asked,

"What mantra do the three of you chant?"

All three of the saints were using the same mantra and they revealed it to him. Literally it meant: We are three and you are three.

"This can't be a mantra!" the scholar scolded, laughing derisively. "It doesn't mean anything. It's a made-up mantra and isn't scriptural."

The saints looked at each other in confusion.

"Surely we're foolish," they said. "What should we do?"

"I'll teach you a scriptural mantra," the scholar replied. "Chant this mantra regularly each day."

So the scholar taught them a new mantra.

After he had instructed them, he said good-bye and sailed away in his ship.

The three saints chanted their new mantra immediately and with great determination. But about fifteen days later one of the saints opened his eyes. He had totally forgotten every word of the new mantra and was once more chanting his old one. He asked his fellow saints,

"Please teach me again the new mantra that the scholar taught. I've forgotten it."

But the others had forgotten it, too, and were once again chanting their old one.

"Oh, Lord," they prayed, certain they were in the wrong by forgetting the mantra, "We're foolish, begging trifling things from You. But please forgive us and bless us so that we don't make this mistake again."

Then the three saints stood up and ran toward the ocean, certain they needed to find the scholar and be taught the mantra again.

When they came to the ocean they kept running. Since they had never left the island, they didn't have a boat. When their feet touched the water, however, they were so engrossed in their determination to catch the scholar that they didn't notice whether it was ground or water beneath their feet. They just kept running.

These saints had no idea that in the yogic scriptures there's a description of the yogic power of walking on water. How could one who has never heard of miraculous powers ever strive to demonstrate them?

Many men and women were standing on the ship's deck. Suddenly they saw the three saints running hand-in-hand across the water toward the ship. The spectators shouted with excitement.

Hearing the commotion, the scholar, who was below the deck came upstairs to investigate. As he approached the ship's edge, he saw the three saints running on the surface of the water. His astonishment knew no bounds when he realized that the very saints whom he had called foolish had this extraordinary yogic power.

Soon the three saints reached the ship and spotted the scholar standing on the deck. Jubilant upon seeing him, they came close to him and prayed humbly,

"Dear scholar, we foolish ones have forgotten your scriptural mantra and have come to bother you again."

Moved by their humility, devotion, and innocence the scholar humbly replied,

"Compassionate saints, I'm glad you've graced me with your darshan again and I bow down to you. Just as there is energy in the mantra, there's energy in your faith. Your devotion to the Lord is the best of all mantras. You have absolutely no need for a new mantra. Just go on chanting your old mantra."

Their problem solved, the innocent saints turned and headed for their island in the same manner in which they had come.

When cold water is put into a boiler, no energy is produced. But when water and fire are used together, steam is produced. Similarly when mantra chanting and devotion are used together they unlock the power inherent in the mantra.

Story #74

*For spiritual progress you must take up your abode in an ashram
every now and then and do spiritual practices. The Guru's house
is your house. It's the abode of peace and happiness, the school of
abstinence and the biggest pilgrimage of knowledge. It's the house
of the Lord. Only a lit lamp can light an unlit lamp. The guru is
the lit lamp and the disciple is the unlit lamp. Even if we study the
scriptures, we can't comprehend certain portions of the scriptures
through our rational mind alone. We need the help of the Sadguru.
The lineage of sacred knowledge continues in this way.*

From the State Assembly to the Saint Assembly

ONCE A VIRTUOUS NONATTACHED saint was wandering
through the countryside. He arrived at an ashram located
near a large city. It was customary for the inhabitants of
this city to visit the ashram daily so they could have the audience
of various saints.

One day the Chief Minister of the city happened to visit and had
the audience of this saint, who was unfamiliar to him. Impressed
by the holy man, the Chief Minister eagerly invited him to attend
the minister's state assembly. Overwhelmed with love the saint
accepted the offer.

The saint made an impressive appearance and the King said
with gratitude,

"Oh, Compassionate One! For a long time now I've enjoyed
the infinite blessings of innumerable great saints who have purified
my state assembly with their holy feet."

The saint was silent and somewhat serious.

Sensing the saint was hesitant to speak, the King humbly
entreated.

"Oh, Gracious One! When you heard my statement, you became serious. I sense that although you wish to say something,

you're hesitant. I have complete faith in your holy feet. I consider you my relative and will listen to whatever you say."

"Oh, King," the saint replied. "I'm pleased with your humility. I don't totally agree with your statement, however, that innumerable great men have purified your assembly."

The King was surprised.

"Why don't you agree?" The King inquired innocently.

"There are some great men who shouldn't be invited to the state assembly," the saint answered. "It's more appropriate to have their darshan where they reside. I'm certain that many great men have come to visit you and honor you as a King at your state assembly. But the great men to whom I refer are extraordinarily unique. They see both king and paupers as equals and are considered to be extremely rare great men. To have their darshan, one should visit them at their saint assembly. You can bring home water from the Ganges in a pot, but the river itself can't be brought home. To drink and bathe fully in the Ganges, you should go to the river itself. At home you can only have the benefit of what you fetched."

To move from worldly consciousness, the state assembly, to divine consciousness, the saint assembly, it's helpful whenever possible to immerse ourselves totally in an environment of love, peace, and higher knowledge, that is, to drink and bathe fully in the Ganges, you should go to the river itself. Examples may be living in the presence of a holy person, attending spiritual retreats, or living in an ashram or a spiritual community.

STORY #75

Beginning spiritual seekers aren't given condensed, terse teachings as they can't properly contemplate or integrate them. For this reason great acharyas give lengthy explanations to beginners and terse teachings to advanced students devoted only to yoga practice. The elaborate teachings for beginning practictioners are provided in the Vedas, Upanishads, Darshans, Puranas, and other true scriptures. The terse teachings for advanced seekers are given in the Brahma Sutras, Yoga Sutras, Narad Bhakti Sutras, and other true scriptures.

THE TEACHINGS OF LORD BRAHMA

ONCE UPON A TIME three yoga sadhaks named Devendra, Danavendra, and Manavendra had a meeting to contemplate life. They were discussing character faults.

First Devendra gave his philosophy.

"We continually make mistakes in life, but since mistakes are often subtle or concealed, they're often invisible. Our eyes allow us to observe everyone but ourselves. To observe ourselves we need a mirror. Only then can we observe our own behavior and change."

Next Manavendra gave his philosophy.

"The genuine guru has pristine vision and can clearly see his disciple's vices and virtues. We should seek help at the divine feet of the Sadguru."

Next Danavendra gave his philosophy.

"Yes, we should go to Lord Brahma, himself, the father of the universe. He's our well-wisher, father, and Sadguru."

They all agreed that the last idea was the best one.

They went to Lord Brahma and presented themselves humbly at his feet. After bowing down and offering their pranams, they sat down in front of him.

Lord Brahma had seen the three coming from a distance and he was pleased. Smiling, and with great tenderness, he asked,

"My sons, are you happy?"

"Yes," Devendra replied softly, "Due to your grace, we're happy. Yet today there's confusion in our hearts, so we've come to you for your teachings."

Lord Brahma was omniscient. He knew what was bothering each of them and he knew they each perceived the root problem differently according to their understanding. With hardly a pause, he uttered his instruction.

"Da," he said. His instruction was merely a single syllable.

As he said the syllable, he gave each seeker a glance, the meaning of which was clear.

"Each of you has a different question for me and I'm responding to each of you individually even though my answer to all three of you is the same."

The three had come to Lord Brahma for instruction, not to debate with him. Thus, when they heard his answer, they were totally satisfied. They looked at each other and then bowed to Lord Brahma. When they stood up to leave, they spoke in unison.

"By your grace, our questions have been resolved."

Devendra interpreted da to mean daman or to suppress. He imagined that in heaven people drank liquor while watching beautiful women dance. He concluded that people shouldn't act this way. They should practice daman, instead. In other words to correct our character faults we should suppress, or check, our bad habits.

Danavendra interpreted da to mean daya or compassion. He concluded that violence is an expression of strong, cruel, ferocious demons within. If we practice compassion our cruelty will diminish.

Manavendra interpreted da to mean dana or charity. He concluded that people who hoard their possessions become demonic in nature. If we practice charity we can avoid accumulating too many possessions and cease acting like animals.

We're all travelers on the same path, so your questions are mine as well. The only difference between us is that I've traveled a little more and some of my questions have been resolved. Thus, the solutions I've found can be useful to you. If our root problem can be resolved, then many questions surrounding it can also be resolved. Our root problems are usually caused by our personal limitations, that is, by our character faults.

STORY #76

Once Lord Buddha conducted an experiment in diet. He began by taking a handful of rice and counting the grains. He then decreased the number of grains he ate each day by one grain. Eventually only one grain remained so he only ate one grain of rice that day. However, one day he fell unconscious from weakness. On that day he decided to take the middle path saying, "If the strings of an instrument are kept too loose, they can't produce music, and if they're kept too tight they'll break. An instrument can only give music when tuned the middle way, neither too loose nor too tight. Similarly the food we eat should be moderate, neither too much nor too little."

Moderation in diet, mitahar, is one of the foundations of spiritual progress. It means to eat the precise amount of food required to keep the body alert and efficient. This isn't easy. Even a wise man can become a fool when eating. Each meal tests our power of discrimination.

MY FORTY-DAY FAST

WHEN I WAS ONLY nineteen years old my Reverend Gurudev gave me mantra initiation. I was required to fast solely on water for forty days. To this day, I can't image how I managed to fast for forty days. I truly believe that I managed only by the grace of my Gurudev. Prior to that time I used to eat two meals and two snacks a day and I would never turn down extra snacks, either.

"From tomorrow onward you should eat only twice a day, "Gurudev told me, giving me preliminary instructions.

I became depressed just hearing this order. My appetite was notorious. Often I would get up in the morning and resolve: "I'll fast today, for sure!" But the moment I spoke those words my appetite would voraciously attack me and I would eat twice as much breakfast and earlier than usual, as well.

"Guruji," I pleaded, "How will I ever be able to eat only twice a day?"

But he didn't change his mind. For the first week I struggled, but then gradually my mind got used to it. For two months I did this and then he changed the routine again.

"After tomorrow, you should eat only once a day and that meal should be moderate."

"I have to eat moderately and only once a day?" I begged.

"Yes," he nodded.

The next week was difficult. But then once again my mind got used to the routine. Gurudev insisted that I eat with him and he informed the sister who served us that I must eat moderately. After I ate the moderate portions she had served, Gurudev would order me to leave the table.

Sometimes the sister cried in pity at my situation. Although we were both required to obey, it was obvious that Gurudev's orders contained no trace of cruelty or oppression. They were full of powerful, tender affection.

Then after keeping me on the dietary regimen of one meal a day, Gurudev instructed that I only drink milk for three months. During the first few days, I felt discomfort again, but afterwards things went fine.

Eventually, Gurudev said,

"My son, starting tomorrow you should fast for forty days and practice mantra japa."

His first two words, "My son," were so sweet and had the power to lessen the bitterness of the task ahead.

Expressing my worry in an amusing way, I repeated to Gurudev a traditional saying: "The face of the compassionate Lord doesn't look upon the hungry person." Then I added, "But when I fast, He'll have to look at me because I'm going to chant mantra japa constantly. And before I chant, I'm going to call upon the Lord and demand that He sit with me for forty days."

"Let the Lord worry about His own helplessness," Gurudev replied with a smile. "Don't do His worrying for Him. Since you've quoted a traditional saying, I'll quote to you from scripture: the word upvas or fasting, is composed of two syllables; up meaning near or close to, and vas meaning to reside. That is, to live close to the Lord. Thus, the Lord sits near the fasting devotee who is helpless with love. Actually a devotee is hungry only for love and since the Lord loves to look with unblinking eyes at the face of the love-hungry devotee, He never leaves him alone."

Finally it was the day of the fast. Guruji initiated me with the mantra and showed me the room where I was to fast.

"You must fast and do mantra japa for forty days," he said. "There's a water pot inside. Every day I'll lock your door from the outside and keep the keys with me. You're free to come for darshan twice a day."

"Guruji," I said, expressing mental anguish and confusion, "Must you bother to lock and unlock the door yourself?"

"Yes," he said with finality. "I'll do this myself."

Such affection for his disciple. What unparalleled grace! I've never been proud of my arduous austerities, not even in a dream. It's all truly due to the divine grace of my Gurudev. He was a great man. I believe he knew me inside and out, and I had unflinching faith in his divine wisdom. I may have had the willpower to fast on water for two or three days, but I know that to fast for forty days was far beyond my capacity.

Thus, on the first day of the fast I bowed to my Gurudev's feet and humbly said,

"Gurudev, fasting forty days is too hard for me. But with your grace, I'll try."

Placing his holy hands on my head he said,

"I bless you," and I felt an energy transmitted into my body. He also gave me comforting guidance:

"My son," he said. "The first three days will be difficult for you, but this discomfort will diminish by the fifth day. By the seventh day you'll have no difficulty at all."

And that's what happened. On the fortieth day of the fast, I was still able to walk. Although there was some physical weakness, I experienced physical alertness and mental joy. I also sat regularly for japa.

Gurudev was very loving to me. Even today when I think back, I feel that he loves me most of all. Whenever this thought comes to me, I lose consciousness. I know for sure that whatever I've received in this world is because of his grace. To me, he is life itself. He means everything to me. By his grace I was able to finish the forty-day fast with no difficulty.

Just as a railroad car can say, "I move only by the grace of the locomotive, only the locomotive has the power to move a railroad car like me." So, too, we move forward by the grace of the guru. Great souls in the past who have experienced the grace of God or Guru have been able to utter only one sentence: "Grace is indescribable."

STORY #77

*People select saints according to their own temperament. One
person likes a scholar, one a renunciate, another an ascetic, another
a yogi, another a devotional saint. Those who worship knowledge,
consider what is said, rather than who is speaking. Those who
worship character, consider who is speaking, rather than what is
said. We can evaluate saints according to their inner and outer
characteristics, but it's important to know that people are often led
astray by outer characteristics.*

THE KING AND THE THREE FAMOUS SAINTS

ONCE UPON A TIME there were three famous saints in
India. One of them had the best reputation of all. A
certain king learned of these saints. The king was a lover
of saints and religion and had the darshan of each of these saints
whenever he could.

"Please be gracious," the king often begged the three saints.
"Visit me often and sanctify my city whenever I extend an
invitation."

"We will definitely come whenever we have a chance," the
saints replied sincerely, giving the king their promise.

One day the king invited the three saints to a special event.
His beloved daughter, the princess, was going to be married. All
three saints accepted the invitation.

On the appointed day, the saints arrived. The king and his
subjects welcomed the saints with pomp and ceremony and gave
each one their own room in the palace. The entire city was full of
love and holy vibrations as the saints gave satsang and discourses
and chanted and sang bhajans.

The saints said they would stay for only four days. On the last
day, the king invited them to dine with him. After the luncheon,
the king paid homage to the first saint and offered him 10,000
golden coins.

"Your Highness, I'm nonattached," the first saint said. "I've accepted only the wealth of the Lord's name and have renounced all other riches. I can't use this gift."

The second saint was sitting nearby. He was extremely famous, the highest saint in India, and he immediately blurted out,

"Reverend saint, give me the gift if you don't want it."

"Take it if you wish," the first saint said.

The second saint accepted the gift, as well as his own gift of 10,000 coins.

The king then offered 10,000 gold coins to the third saint.

"Please forgive me, Your Highness," the third saint said. "I have no need for wealth. Spiritual practices are my wealth. I can't use this currency."

Again the famous second saint spoke up.

"Give the gift to me if you don't need it."

The third saint consented so now the second saint had 30,000 gold coins.

The king was astonished. He couldn't imagine why this great saint was so fond of wealth. Although he didn't like this conduct, he remained silent. He was extremely impressed by the sacrifice of the first and third saints and extremely disappointed with the second saint. Nevertheless, he respectfully bid farewell to all three saints.

Ten years passed.

The king decided to make a pilgrimage with many of his subjects. On the day of departure, a thousand pilgrims set forth. In order to handle emergencies and carry supplies the king provided chariots, carts, horses, camels, and elephants.

Two weeks later the pilgrims arrived in Kashi, the city of Lord Vishwanath.

"Victory to the Lord!" The tired people joyfully proclaimed.

Needing an inn for the king and his staff, the king's attendants made inquiries and learned of a huge inn nearby called, Maharaj Ratnasinhji Chauhan.

The king was curious when he heard this, for he himself was named Ratnasinhji Chauhan. Yet he had never visited Kashi before. He was especially interested in finding out the name of the Maharaja who had built this inn.

When the king approached the inn he was further surprised to read the inscription written over the entrance door. It said:

"This is the inn of Maharaj Ratnasinhji Chauhan of Devagiri."

He himself was the king of Davagiri! Was this his own inn?

Thoroughly puzzled, he led the procession into the inn. The innkeeper graciously made every kind of arrangement for the pilgrims' comfort. They were extremely pleased with their accommodations.

The king then approached the innkeeper and asked,

"Who commissioned this inn and when was it built?"

"Ten years ago Siddha Babaji was the invited guest of the King of Devagiri," the innkeeper replied. "It was for the marriage ceremony of the king's daughter. The king gave him 30,000 gold coins as dakshina. The inn was funded by this spiritual offering."

The king was flabbergasted, for he now understood the greatness of this high saint. He realized that the saint had practiced inner, rather than outer manifestation of his saintliness. Ten years ago the saint had said nothing, not wanting to reveal how he would use this gift to serve humanity.

High saints don't have the desire to exhibit their virtues. Good men try to hide their virtues and bad men try to hide their vices. But neither virtue nor vice can be hidden. How can one conceal the perfume of flowers in a beautiful garden, or the putrid smell of a rotten corpse in a ditch? May God grant us the strength to become saintly and to recognize a saint.

STORY #78

The Lord's play, or maya, is totally beyond our grasp. I'm surprised that I, accustomed to living within the four walls of my residence in India, have suddenly come to America. The strong force of your love has brought me here. My only purpose in coming is to meet my grandchildren. I haven't come to spread yoga or religion. To me in fact this whole visit seems like a dream or the Lord's maya. Once Lord Shri Krishna showed this maya to his childhood friend, Sudama, who had pleaded to see it. That's the purpose of this story.

SUDAMA AND THE LORD'S MAYA

ONE DAY, THE AFFECTIONATE Lord Krishna said, "I haven't seen my childhood friend, Sudama, for a long time. If I call him here to me, he won't feel relaxed and friendly with me, because I'm a King and he's still mortal."

So Lord Krishna decided to go to Sudama's home.

Calling for His ministers, he declared,

"I'm going on a secret journey and will return in a few days."

Sudama was a humble devotee of the Lord. His home was small. As a devotee dear to Shri Krishna, Sudama had voluntarily accepted poverty. He was content to live in this state because it helped him pray to the Lord with a humble heart.

"Dear Lord," he often prayed, "if you want to come to this house, come in simple dress and live here like me in quiet simplicity. All I want to be is a devotee. I don't want wealth and luxury. You can pray in that corner of my house, and I will pray in this corner. There isn't a single sweet snack to even look at in my house, let alone eat. Sometimes we pray for two or three days pass while living only on yawns."

So, as twilight settled over Sudama's house, Lord Krishna, dressed in simple peasant clothes, knocked on Sudama's door.

Sudama was seated in meditation and his wife was busy with housework. On hearing the knock, his wife set aside her work and opened the door.

"Sister," said Krishna. "I've sneaked away to see you and Sudama and would like to stay here for a few days."

Sudama's wife recognized the visitor as Rajayogi Lord Krishna, her husband's only true friend in the world. She was overwhelmed with joy and welcomed him with love.

Krishna washed his face and hands in a basin of water and then sat comfortably on a ragged mat in the courtyard. He took a sip of water from a jug Sudama's wife had placed beside him.

"Sister," he said. "Your water here is even better than that of Dwarka."

"Yes," she said, smiling. "What you say is true, because Dwarka's water isn't water; it's nectar. It isn't simply sweet; it's ultra sweet, because you turn water into nectar wherever you live. After drinking nectar all the time, it's only natural that the water of a friend's house would taste different."

"Sister," replied Lord Krishna, "My brother has taught you a lot. Thank you. Are you going to serve me something to eat?"

"Rice and beans with curry and spinach."

"My favorite food!"

Just then Sudama opened the door of his meditation room. His delight knew no bounds at the sight of his friend Shri Krishna sitting in his courtyard. Embracing each other warmly, the two friends let tears of love flow unabashedly from their eyes. Over and over, Sudama murmured,

"Shri Krishna...Shri Krishna...Shri Krishna."

And again and again, Shri Krishna exclaimed,

"Sudama...Sudama...Sudama."

These weren't just words. They were streams of pure love flowing between two united hearts.

Then the two old friends began to talk. When it was time to eat, they continued talking right through dinner. They would eat a little and then talk. Then eat a little more and talk some more. For hours they were oblivious of time. Even after going to bed, they kept talking and talking.

Midnight came and Sudama's wife reminded her husband,

"Our brother has traveled a long way by a secret route. Only the Lord Himself knows how he reached here. He must be tired, so let him rest for a while."

But Lord Krishna objected.

"Sister," he said. "Go to bed and rest peacefully. Although I'm a King, you've forgotten that I'm also a shepherd. My job is to care for the cows. This requires running to and fro all day long. I've climbed up and down Mount Govardhan many times in just one day. So my body isn't weakened by this ordinary trip. My friend, Sudama, though is a Brahmin who spends the whole day reading scriptures and praying to the Lord. If Sudama walked just to the outskirts of the village he would be tired, so he may need rest, not me. Anyway, I've been dreaming of seeing Sudama again, and I can tell you that the only reason I went to sleep every night was so that I could dream about him. Now that I'm here with him, face to face, sleep won't come. So please go to bed and let us talk."

And so the two friends talked all night and neither one slept.

The next day, Lord Krishna played for hours with his little nephew and niece. He bounced them on his lap and their laughing voices echoed through the house.

On the third day the two friends set out for a nearby lake. As they walked, Sudama reflected to himself:

"Shri Krishna is a raja yogi. The rishi munis consider him to be the incarnation of Lord Vishnu himself. They say that his maya is incredible. Now that he's right here with me, why shouldn't I take advantage of this opportunity and have a look?

So Sudama said,

"I want to see your maya, Shri Krishna. Please show me!"

Lord Krishna smiled.

"Don't talk that way. My maya isn't worth seeing."

"Please don't turn me down! I'm your best friend. It isn't right that I should go without seeing it."

"If you keep on talking like this, we'll be late for dinner," Lord Krishna said.

Before they had left for the lake, Sudama's wife had told them: "Remember that the meal is almost ready, so don't take long. The only thing left for me to do is to roll the chappatis. I'll wait until you come back for that, so they'll remain hot for you."

But Sudama persisted in his request to Lord Krishna.

"Forget the chappatis," he said. "Tell me right now, are you going to show me your maya or not?"

"I'm not opposed to revealing my maya to you," replied Lord Krishna, "I only hesitate because I'm afraid you'll regret the experience."

"I want to find out for myself," said Sudama.

"Alright, then I'll reveal it to you."

Sudama smiled in anticipation. By now they had reached the lake and were preparing to bathe. They walked into the water and then Lord Krishna said,

"Sudama, how long can you hold your breath under water? Let's have a contest."

"But brother," stammered Sudama. "You're a raja yogi. I'm just a novice devotee. You can surely hold your breath longer than I."

"No buts," Krishna said.

"Then let's at least experiment first," Sudama said. "We'll both dive together."

"All right," Lord Krishna replied.

They stood in deeper water facing each other and then went under together. Sudama came up first. When he came up, Lord Krishna was gone.

"Where has Shri Krishna gone?" He said, looking around. There were lots of people walking along the shore. "I know we both went under together."

He waited for a few minutes, but Lord Krishna was nowhere in sight.

He left the water and noticed with great surprise that he was standing on an unfamiliar beach in some unknown city. When he realized he was lost, he stopped a few people and asked for directions back to his hometown.

"How far is my hometown from here?" He asked each one.

"Brother," they all said. "I've never heard of such a place. How could I tell you how far it is from here?"

After some time, he had no choice but to settle down in that city. Eventually he forgot his wife and children. Since he had to work to make a living, he engaged himself in an occupation and eventually achieved some success. He married and raised a family.

In that city people observed a special custom upon the death of a married woman. Her husband was cremated along with her body.

One day Sudama's wife suddenly died. His neighbors grabbed him and took him to the funeral pyre so he wouldn't run away. But Sudama had no intention of being cremated. Using his wits, he quickly devised a plan.

"The lake is nearby," he told his captors. "Would you let me bathe in it before you proceed with my funeral?"

The people consented, so Sudama walked into the lake. Dwelling on the name of the Lord, he dove into the lake, held his breath, and swam away as far as he could. When he couldn't hold his breath any longer, he popped his head out of the water. His face was full of fear, hoping he had swum far from the funeral site.

To his great surprise, however, Lord Krishna was standing right next to him.

"Shri Krishna!" Sudama cried, throwing his arms around Lord Krishna.

"Sudama?" Lord Krishna said. "Why are you looking so terrified?"

"Shouldn't I be terrified? They're going to cremate me with my dead wife!"

"Sudama! What kind of crazy talk is that? Your wife is back home in the kitchen. Where's this funeral you're talking about and where are these people?"

Sudama stared completely baffled at Lord Krishna's face. Then he stammered,

"Then what on earth did I see? Oh, Krishna! Don't ever show me your maya again."

"Oh, come on!" Lord Krishna teased. "Just one more time!"

"No, brother, no! For God's sake, don't show it to me again!"

"Then let's go home now. Your wife is waiting for us. And we'll be right on time for dinner, too. Your swim lasted only six minutes."

"I lived fifty years in six minutes? I tell you, brother, your maya is totally extraordinary."

Everything we perceive is the Lord's maya. It's our great fortune just to be able to say a few prayers to Him. This world is an ocean of pain and it's sheer foolishness to try to find happiness in it. The Lord alone is the ocean of bliss. We must worship Him and accept any pain we encounter as being His grace. Hold tightly to the mantra and believe with your whole heart that you are clinging to the holy feet of the Lord.

STORY #79

*Stealing was considered an art in ancient times, a form of enter-
tainment, never to be used as a vocation but simply as a game.
Contests were arranged for clever people to demonstrate their
skills. If a theft couldn't be solved, the king would issue a procla-
mation of amnesty. The guilty thief would then fearlessly present
himself to the state and disclose the trick he used in committing the
crime. He would be set free and given a reward of gold coins. This
is one such story. I'll tell it to you so that you will know something
about the historical culture of India.*

THE THEFT OF THE CLOTH

ONCE A DISCUSSION TOOK place in a large kingdom on the
art of stealing. As the seminar ended, it was decided that
an expert in the art should be questioned and asked to
demonstrate his skills. The first name that occurred to everyone
was that of a prosperous tailor in town, who was a favorite among
the king's family. After the seminar, the king sent for him and
said,

"Mohanbhai, two days ago, we held a seminar on the art of
stealing. Many participants nominated you as the leading expert
in the art. Is this true?"

"Your Excellency," Mohanbhai replied with dignity, "Having
served your family for many years, I'm naturally quite prosperous.
Let it be clear that I've never stolen anything to acquire wealth,
but I have done so to practice the art. No art can develop without
practice. Stealing is unacceptable if it's done for wealth. It should
be practiced only as an art form."

"It's all right if you want to steal for the sake of the art," the
king replied in a friendly way, "but what would you do if I ordered
you not to steal at all?"

"You're the king," Mohanbhai respectfully replied, "and you
are powerful. I would honor your command. Nevertheless, I'm

an artist, and I must say that I would always get away with a little bit."

"And if I ordered you not to do even a small amount of stealing? Then what?" the king asked.

"Then, I must confess," Mohanbhai said, "that I wouldn't call myself an expert artist if I couldn't steal at least something, anyway."

"Then we'll have to conduct an experiment," the king said. "The princess is about to be married. Many dresses need to be made for the wedding. I'll have you sew the dresses, but you must do so under the watchful eyes of the state inspectors."

"As you desire," Mohanbhai said.

The king ordered the cloth for the dresses. Mohanbhai sat in the palace under the close observation of the inspectors and began sewing the dresses. At the end of each day, the king ordered the inspectors to check Mohanbhai's pockets before he went home.

One day, Mohanbhai's twelve-year-old daughter and eight-year-old son came to the palace. As the two stood at the door, the daughter said loudly,

"Father! My brother won't stay home today. He's very mischievous and bothers everybody."

"Go away!" Mohanbhai shouted angrily at his daughter. "Take him home! Can't you see I'm busy?"

"But he wants five rupees," his daughter said.

"Five rupees!" One of the inspectors said with surprise. "Why does he need so much money? Mohanbhai, I think you've spoiled this child! Otherwise why would this little boy ask for five rupees?"

"Father!" the boy demanded, "Give me five rupees!"

"I didn't bring any money with me," Mohanbhai said. "Go home! Right now! I'll give you some money when I get home."

"No! No! I want rupees now!"

Mohanbhai picked up his wooden tailor's gauge and threw it at his son. He did it hard, but in such a manner as to scare the boy and not to hurt him.

"Are you going home or not?" Mohanbhai shouted

"No! No! I want rupees!" His son shouted back.

Mohanbhai then took off his shoe and threw it in anger at his son.

"This is the only kind of rupee I have!" He hollered. "Now go home!"

The inspector was afraid the child would be injured.

"Mohanbhai," he said, "Don't throw things at your child. He may get hurt."

The boy was unfazed. Keeping the shoe, he hollered back at his father,

"I'll only give you back your shoe if you give me rupees!"

"Oh, really?" Mohanbhai said, unfazed as well at the brashness of his son, "Then take these rupees, too!" And he threw his other shoe at his son.

The two children ran away with the shoes and the inspector burst into laughter.

"Mohanbhai," he said, "Today you'll have to go home barefoot."

"I don't mind," Mohanbhai said. "At least those kids are gone! I can't stand to be disturbed when I'm working. From now on I'm going to keep some stones here to make sure they stay away,"

"Mohanbhai," the inspector said, "Don't keep stones with you. You may hurt the children."

"I know that," Mohanbhai said, "I'll be careful. But I must scold them in this manner or they won't mind me. I must be firm."

When Mohanbhai had finished sewing the dresses for the wedding, the king called the inspectors and said,

"Did you watch him carefully to make sure there was no stealing?"

"Yes, your Excellency," the inspectors said. "We checked his pockets every day before he went home. We're sure he didn't steal a thing."

Then the king called Mohanbhai.

"Well, Mohanbhai," the king said, "Have you succeeded in your art or failed?"

"By your grace, I've succeeded," Mohanbhai said, taking out some cloth.

The king was pleased.

"You're truly an expert at this art," the king said. "How did you steal the cloth?"

"If you're pleased with my skill," Mohanbhai said, "Promise me a reward of 25,000 rupees in addition to my regular wage for sewing the dresses. Then I'll disclose my secret."

The king agreed.

Mohanbhai described the whole incident with his two children and said that he had hidden the cloth in both shoes!

The king's face lit up with a smile.

STORY #80

*When our only aim is to attain the Supreme Being, nonattachment
in its final form is accomplished spontaneously without effort. Just
as a traveler heading west is naturally going away from the east,
a seeker heading toward liberation is naturally moving away from
worldly illusion. When seekers desiring liberation begin yoga
sadhana, previous attachments remaining in their minds, however
few, manifest and create disturbance. But the seeker frees himself
from them through the power of discrimination, which increases
daily as his mind and body purify. The more our love for the Lord
increases, the more our love for worldly illusion decreases.*

THE NONATTACHED YOGI BHATRIHARI

ONCE UPON A TIME in ancient India there was a valiant
king named, Bhatrihari. Even today he's regarded as
one of the best Sanskrit poets and yogis. His kingdom,
Ujjayini, still remains a place of pilgrimage.

After he renounced his throne, Bhatrihari practiced yoga sadhana for a long time and finally achieved samadhi. The great yogis
who have achieved this union with God truly personify the practice of nonattachment. Some of them wear only a loincloth. Their
nonattachment has blossomed to such an extent that they detach
their consciousness from their body and mind and reside solely in
the soul.

One day the great yogi Bhatrihari came to a cemetery while
traveling. When he sat down to rest under a canopy of trees, he
noticed that the bark loincloth he was wearing was torn in several
places.

"This needs to be sewn," he thought.

So he stood up and searched around until he found two thorns.
He used one thorn to make a hole in the end of the other. But
when he tried to thread his crude needle with fiber from the bark

of a tree, he was unable to see well enough in the fast-approaching twilight.

At that moment, Lord Shiva was traveling across the sky with Mother Parvati. Bhatrihari was chanting as he was trying to thread the needle.

"Oh namah Shivaya. Om namah Shivaya. Om namah Shivaya," he chanted sweetly over and over with great devotion.

It was his usual practice to chant like this while performing any task. The words of the chant fell upon the ears of Mother Parvati and she looked down and spotted Bhatrihari. Mother Parvati was a perfect devotee of Lord Shiva and she loved Shiva's devotees as much as she loved Shiva himself. For this reason she desired to meet Bhatrihari.

"My Lord," Mother Parvati humbly asked, "One of your devotees is sitting alone under a tree. Please come down to earth with me. I would like to meet him."

"He's not worth meeting," Lord Shiva replied.

"But he's one of your perfect devotees!" Exclaimed Mother Parvati with surprise. "How can you say he's not worth meeting?"

The omniscient Lord Shiva thought for awhile. He knew what he had said was correct, but he also knew that Mother Parvati didn't understand his statement. So he changed his mind.

"Come on, then," he said, and he and Mother Parvati landed on the earth.

They approached Bhatrihari and stood behind him, but Mother Parvati wasn't satisfied.

"I want to see his face," she said.

"Move closer, then," Lord Shiva whispered. "Say whatever you want to him."

"Bhatrihari, my son," Mother Parvati said. "I'm Parvati, your mother. I've come down to earth with your father, Lord Shiva, to meet you. We're both standing behind you."

Bhatrihari didn't reply. He didn't even turn his head. He simply kept sewing.

Mother Parvati found his behavior strange, in fact, rude. She rebuked him saying,

"It was my wish to come down to earth just to meet you. Yet you won't even turn around to look at me?"

"Don't talk so much," Bhatrihari said kindly. He wasn't mad. "Have you grown so old that you don't remember anything?" Every word he spoke was filled with tender love for Mother Parvati and this pleased her heart.

"It's true that I've grown old," Mother Parvati said. "But I don't believe you when you say I don't remember anything."

"You've forgotten the most important thing," Bhatrihari said. "Aren't you everywhere? In front of me? Behind me? Above me? Beneath me? You're everywhere, remember? You're in my heart, in my sight, in my speech. So how can I believe you when you tell me that you're standing behind me? I can see you even in the hole in this thorn and in the fiber of this bark. Why should I turn around to see you when you're right here in front of me?"

Mother Parvati's heart opened with love. Now she understood the words of Lord Shiva when he said that Bhatrihari wasn't worth meeting. She already knew him!

"My son," she said with affection, "I'm pleased with you. Ask any boon you want."

"You're talking nonsense again," Bhatrihari said with indifference. He didn't even turn around as he spoke. "But all right, if you insist on granting me a boon, take this thorn and thread it for me. How can I disobey your order?"

Mother Parvati threaded the thorn with the fiber and then expressed her sadness.

"Don't you want anything else from me?" She asked.

"Just go away and don't bother me," Bhatrihari replied, again with great tenderness. "The fact that I've attained you is the greatest boon you could give me. I don't believe that a greater boon exists in this world. You are boons and boons are you. What happiness can I possible receive from any other boon?"

This kind of nonattachment is the nonattachment of great yogis. When we begin our spiritual journey we must start from a state of high attachment and gradually travel in the direction of nonattachment. We can practice sadhana only according to our capacity. Start by performing simple acts of service for others. Nonattachment grows whenever we perform selfless actions. When a schoolteacher solves a math problem on the blackboard, does he solve it for himself? No, he solves it for his students. Any action not motivated by selfish desire, performed for the love of God, is the best of all forms of nonattachment.

STORY #81

We can fulfill many ordinary desires within a day, a month, or a year. But to fulfill extraordinary desires, we must strive for innumerable lifetimes. A weak obstacle can destroy a weak thought, but even the greatest obstacle can't destroy a bhavana, a strong thought, or strong conviction. When we use mantra to feed our thoughts we create an ocean of energy and strength.

THE SQUIRREL AND THE BRIDGE

IN THE ANCIENT ALLEGORY of the Ramayan, when Lord Ram received the news from courageous Hanuman that Sita had been kidnapped by Ravan, the king of Lanka, and that she was being kept in Ashoka Vana, he immediately decided to invade Lanka.

Ram's army of monkeys came to the ocean and at once began building a bridge to cross it. A squirrel living nearby watched the huge army of monkeys arriving. She observed them for awhile and soon discovered that there was one special man among them. Each morning the entire army would pay their respects to him by bowing down. Afterwards they would begin their daily task of building the bridge

One day the squirrel received the audience of that great man. She developed a feeling in her heart of deep love and felt a desire to serve him. Since the bridge building seemed an act of service to this great man, she willingly joined in the task.

The squirrel carefully observed how the monkeys were constructing the bridge. Before the monkeys moved each of the large rocks needed for the bridge, they would chant the name of Ram and the rock would float on the water. Because she didn't have the strength to lift the huge rocks, the squirrel was sad. Yet her strong desire to serve gave birth to an idea.

She went close to the bridge and happily began rolling in the sand on the seashore. Each time she performed this action, sand would stick to her fur. Then she would place all the sand between the large rocks on the bridge. She would make twenty or thirty trips with sand in the same amount of time that it took a monkey to place one rock on the bridge.

When the monkeys saw her loving, eager service, they were all so moved that they forgot the difficulty of their own labor and hurried to bring the rocks to the bridge. The tiny squirrel had soon inspired the entire army to work more efficiently.

Thus, the monkeys felt that the squirrel had deeper devotion for Ram than they did. They perceived her true love and received more joy from observing her devotion than from the devotion in their own hearts. The strength of our devotion will determine whether it manifests partially or totally. True devotion is always total, no matter how it's displayed.

Soon the sun set and the monkeys stopped their work. Night came and the entire army of monkeys bowed to Lord Ram and sat in front of him. Many of the monkeys were eager to talk about the squirrel's loving service, but they sat silently and looked at the courageous Hanuman for permission to speak. The squirrel was also in silent attendance. Hiding herself at the feet of Hanuman so that no one could see her, she gazed continuously and rapturously at Lord Ram. Naturally the wise Hanuman knew what she was up to, but acted as if nothing was happening.

"Lord," said one monkey eagerly, "Today a tiny squirrel destroyed the sense of ego in our devotion to you. We were carrying huge rocks and she was carrying sand. She continually rolled in the sand on the seashore so that sand stuck to her. She brought the sand to the bridge and placed it between the large stones. In the time we took to bring one rock, she had brought twenty or thirty loads of sand. We experienced boundless joy today at the sight of her loving service."

After hearing this tale, Lord Ram expressed his happiness at the squirrel's service. Suddenly, Hanuman gently picked up the squirrel and lovingly placed her at the feet of the Lord. All the monkeys shouted with joy. The gracious Lord stroked her tiny body. His fingers left impressions on her fur. It was as if the unseen grace of the Lord had become visible.

Like the squirrel, we're all tiny seekers. Even if we can't attain enough nonattachment to carry big boulders, we'll definitely progress if we carry a bit of sand. Nonattachment is extremely patient and tolerant. It's been standing outside the door of our mind for many lifetimes. It will enter whenever we call it and then the dawn of knowledge, devotion, and yoga will break. As seekers, we're all trying to build a bridge, across the ocean of maya to God. At first we don't even know that Soul bliss exists, but then we see others striving for it and devotion is born. In the end like the squirrel it's our devotion not our worthiness that finds favor with God, and the gracious Lord strokes us with His grace.

STORY #82

*Lord Krishna says in the Bhagavad Gita, to control the mind and
to control the wind is the same. Extraordinary seekers understand
the importance of mental steadiness. They take immediate steps to
calm their minds before they enter their meditation room.*

THE MAN WHO RESCUED A DOG

ONCE UPON A TIME during the monsoon season a well-
known, dignified gentleman set out for his morning
walk. He happened upon a dog stuck in the thick mud of
a ditch. The dog was unable to free itself. The man paused, studied the painful situation, and then jumped into the muddy ditch
without giving a thought for his fine, clean clothes.

The frightened dog was struggling violently to extricate itself.
Its eyes were rolling wildly with terror. As the man approached,
the dog bared its teeth, snarled and snapped. When the man pulled
on the animal to free it, the dog bit the man's hand.

The man's only thought, however, was to free the dog. There
was no anger in his mind. In spite of the pain in his hand he continued to tug. Finally after great effort, he freed the dog from the
mud.

When the man climbed out of the ditch, his entire body and
clothes were soaked with mud. He walked home casually, not the
least bit embarrassed to be in public in such a dirty condition.

When his friends heard about the rescue they were impressed.

"That was a wonderful thing you did," they said. "You saved
that poor animal. We respect you for what you did."

"No," the man said, shrugging off the compliment. "I don't de-
serve such praise. I didn't rescue the dog for the reasons you think.
I actually did it for me. When I saw the dog suffering in the ditch,
I was so heartbroken that I rescued him just to sooth my troubled
mind. I was merely helping myself. Had I returned home without

rescuing the dog, I would have felt guilty for months. Saving the dog was a greater favor to myself than the animal."

Before we enter our meditation room, we should attend to our thoughts first. Are we angry at someone? Are we hurt by something? Do we need to take care of something? The music of the Lord can't be heard on a radio full of static.

STORY #83

Eliminating negative thoughts is a form of tapas which purifies the mind and body. Every thought transmitted is eventually received. A seeker should gather positive thoughts and destroy negative thoughts.

Tapas of the mind involves peace of mind, gentleness, silence, self-control, and purity.

THE STATE FAMILY AND THE SANDALWOOD

ONCE UPON A TIME there was a man named, Buddhidhan. Old Buddhidan was the chief secretary of a large kingdom and he was pleased to hear that his Gurudev had come to the city. Buddhidhan went for darshan and entered the room during satsang. His Gurudev was giving an excellent discourse on the power of thought, especially thoughts of love and hate, and the effects of positive and negative thoughts. Buddhidhan was touched and deeply contemplated the words of his Gurudev.

The next day Buddhidhan had a meeting with the King.

"Chief secretary," the King said, "Tomorrow is our monthly procession day. I would like to have you come along and sit with me to discuss matters of state."

"As you wish, Your Excellency," Buddhidhan said, and the following morning the procession began promptly.

As the King and his entourage traveled through the city, the King spotted the mansion of the richest man in town. With the exception of this mansion, all of the houses lining the street were built exactly the same distance from the road. Because the mansion protruded beyond the others, it slightly distorted the symmetry of the scene.

"Chief secretary," the King said. "The front of this rich man's house protrudes slightly and mars the beauty of this road. Have that part of his house cut off."

"As you wish, Your Excellency," replied Buddhidhan, noting the King's order in his notebook.

At the end of the day, however, old Buddhidhan reflected more deeply upon the King's order.

"These processions have occurred for years and years," he thought to himself, "And that mansion was built many years ago. This slight ugliness isn't new. Why did the King wait so long to mention it? Moreover, this rich man has always been loyal to the King. If he were to find out about the King's remarks today he would be heartbroken. The other night in satsang, my Gurudev said that only a negative thought would provoke negativity in the mind of another. Does this mean that the rich man had a negative thought toward the King today? If not, then what provoked the King to suddenly think ill of this rich man?"

Buddhidhan decided to meet with the rich man privately. He visited him the very next day. The rich man was pleased to see him.

"Chief secretary," the rich man said, welcoming Buddhidhan warmly, "Did you come for a special purpose?"

"Yes," replied Buddhidhan.

"Please tell me, then, what's on your mind?"

"Have you been holding negative thoughts about the King or his family lately?" Asked Buddhidhan.

Somewhat taken back, the rich man said,

"What a strange comment. I'm loyal to the King. I've never even dreamed a negative thought about my King!"

"I have complete faith in your loyalty to the King," said the chief secretary. "Yet, try to remember if you might have had any negative thought at all against the state family."

The rich man thought a long time. Then he remembered that such a thought had indeed occurred.

"Yes," acknowledged the rich man, "Two years ago, I bought a large amount of sandalwood which has remained in storage unsold. Recently while discussing my holdings with my accountant, I noticed how much money I had invested in this sandalwood and yet it remains unsold. At that time the thought occurred to me that if someone in the state family would die, I could be free of this debt." In those days sandalwood caskets were made mainly for members of the state family.

"I'll buy the sandalwood from you," Buddhidhan said, "I'll keep it in storage for use by the state family. That way you can be free of your debt."

"But how did you know that a negative thought had occurred to me?" Asked the rich man perplexed.

"I'll explain that later to you," Buddhidhan said, and then he left.

A month passed.

Once again it was time for the King's monthly procession and once again Buddhidhan accompanied the King. When the procession came to the rich man's mansion, the King remembered his order from a month ago.

"Chief secretary," the King said, "During the last procession, I ordered you to have the protruding part of this rich man's house cut off. Have you given this order to the state officers?"

"No, Your Excellency," replied Buddhidhan. "I've noted the order in my notebook, but I've been busy with state affairs. I haven't had time to carry it out."

"Good," said the King, "I'm glad you haven't given the order yet. Cancel it now. This rich man is loyal to the state and such an order would break his heart."

"Anything you say, Your Excellency," replied Buddhidhan.

Old Buddhidhan knew for sure now that it had been the sandalwood which had provoked negativity in the rich man's mind, for the thought had disappeared from the rich man's mind after he had sold the sandalwood.

The next day, Buddhidhan visited the rich man and related the whole incident to him.

This event has scientific importance and shouldn't be considered a matter of coincidence. Whenever we think either positive or negative thoughts about someone, these thoughts register as either love or hate in that person's mind. To prevent the birth of negative thoughts and to achieve peacefulness, become friends with sexual restraint, moderation in diet, exercise, avoidance of vice, study of scripture, friendship with good persons, observance of rules, dutifulness, determination, affinity for virtuous living, and avoidance of faults. Without these, mental and physical disturbances creep in and mar the path of our spiritual progress.

STORY #84

Nonattachment is one of the five scripturally prescribed goals of spiritual life. It means to not accumulate or hoard. We're born attached so naturally we want to accumulate things. It's as difficult to move from attachment to nonattachment as it is to move from the earth to the sky. It simply can't be done in a single bound. Only a gradually step- by- step ascent is possible. If a thousand pounds of grain were piled in front of us do you think we could eat it all in a day? Of course not. But if we had a hundred years to live we could eat ten piles that big.

THE OLD MAN AND THE MANGO TREE

ONCE THERE WAS A young man named, Kumaril. Kumaril had a garden in the open courtyard of his home. One day as he entered the garden, he saw his elderly uncle, Padmakant, busy at work. As Kumaril came closer, he saw that his uncle was energetically planting seedlings. It was obvious that Padmakant even at the age of ninety, loved to work. Kumaril was impressed by his uncle's industriousness.

"Uncle," Kamaril said respectfully, "What are you planting?"

Padmakant stopped working and looked up at Kumaril smiling,

"My son," he said. "I'm planting mango trees."

Seeing about fifteen small mango plants, Kumaril asked,

"You're planting so many?"

"Only fifteen," Padmakant remarked.

"Don't you think that's too many for this garden?" Kumaril inquired.

"No, it's all right," Padmakant said. "There's no other place to plant them."

"They'll bear lots of mangoes," Kumaril added as a compliment to his uncle.

"Thank you," Padmakant replied. "May that thought come true."

"But uncle," Kumaril said laughing, "You're ninety years old! When will these mango trees bear fruit?"

"In twelve years," Padmakant answered.

"But you may leave your body before then. Why are you doing this work?"

"Son, I'm sure that I'll be home with God before these mango trees bear fruit," said Padmakant. "But I'm planting these trees for others, not for myself. For ninety years, I've eaten mangoes from trees which had been planted by other people. Now I want to plant some mango trees so others may eat from trees I've planted."

STORY #85

A pair of pliers is used to tighten and loosen things and sometimes to straighten things out. Wouldn't it be nice if we had a tool to straighten us out? For that we need the tools of self discipline and right conduct. Right conduct is achieved by right company and right company is achieved by discrimination, that is, by knowing who and what is good for us and who and what isn't good for us.

SEPARATING RICE FROM THE HUSK

O NCE I WAS GIVING lectures on the Gita in a small town. After each talk, I used to go for a walk just to exercise a bit after sitting for so long. One day a lawyer joined me. Soon another lawyer joined us and the two of them started talking about their profession.

Then four or five people joined us. They recognized the two lawyers and they were interested in a particular case. They all talked with great animation for about ten minutes and then the first lawyer turned to me and said,

"Guruji, this is worldly talk. You don't understand any of this. And you talk about God all the time and we don't understand any of that!"

"Are you trying to start an argument?" I asked. He knew I was joking. "Is that why you told me that? Because you're a lawyer, do you want to argue about this?"

"Yes!" he said with a laugh, "Let's argue!"

"Well then, you're wrong!" I said. "You say I don't know anything about the world, but I do. I know plenty about the world, but I've chosen to give the world up. How could I give the world up if I couldn't recognize it? We receive rice only when we separate it from the husk, don't we? But we must know what the husk looks like first so we don't throw away the rice and keep the husk."

He laughed again! He liked that line of reasoning very much!

"You've won!" He said. "For once I have nothing to say."

Keep the company of satsanga, or truth. This will purify your mind and help to separate the rice from the husk. We've accumulated countless wrong thoughts and desires from many incarnations and satsanga will gradually eliminate these thoughts. Only that which can change the direction of our mind can really effect us. Satsanga has the power to do that.

STORY #86

*If we compare our life to a boat, then the guru is the captain or
guide and the world is the ocean. The opposite shore is the Lord.
Those who are having fun on this side, have no need for a guide,
as they are happy where they are. For many years we stay on this
side of the ocean. We go from one illusion to another thinking we
are happy.*

THE INTOXICATED CHOBA

ONCE THERE WAS A gentleman addicted to marijuana. He
didn't smoke it, but he crushed it into a drink. Every
afternoon he crushed it up and then mixed it with water,
milk, and spices to make it tasty and as strong as possible.

He lived in Mathura, a famous pilgrimage place in India. He
was a choba. Chobas are people famous for their extreme weight,
size, and their ability to eat large quantities of food. These people
sometimes drink marijuana, then they eat a lot, and then they
swim in the Jamuna River. Then they get out of the water, drink
more marijuana, eat again, and swim in the river again. They have
tremendous strength and physical power.

One day this gentleman was grinding and grinding his marijuana to make it especially strong. It was twilight time and he
got overly intoxicated. First he got dizzy. Then he started seeing
double. Whenever he looked at someone, he saw two. Then his
legs got rubbery and he couldn't walk properly.

"Come on," his friends finally said, putting their arms around
him and holding him up. "Try to walk straight."

"I'm walking fine!" He said. "There's nothing wrong with
me! You're the ones who don't know how to walk!"

So his friends got discouraged and left him alone.

Later than evening this gentleman decided he would take a
boat across the Jamuna River. It was night, dark outside, and he

was extremely intoxicated. He pushed off in the boat determined to row across the Jamuna River alone.

He was a powerful man. He could row for hours and hours at a time. So he kept on rowing and rowing and rowing, all night long.

Morning came.

As daylight spread across the Jamuna River, the choba slowly began to see things clearly again. The effects of the marijuana had worn off. He was sweaty and tired from rowing all night. His arms ached and his hands were sore from the oars. But much to his surprise, his boat was in the exact same place. In his intoxicated state, he had forgotten to take up the anchor.

We, too, are also under illusion. Our boat is also anchored and we're rowing and rowing, but our boat doesn't move. If we desire to grow spiritually, we have to lift the anchor from our boat and firmly push off toward the other shore. The boat ride is difficult. There are tremendous storms of lust and anger, and great whirlpools of greed and ego, and crocodiles of pride and attachment. These things are so powerful, that if they simply brush against our boat the entire boat rocks and gets turned in the wrong direction. The boat has a cloth sail. The cloth sail is self control. But the great winds of lust and anger tear the sail, and so to complete our journey we must pray to God. Lord, You be my guide. I desire to know You and go to the opposite shore. Lord, You be my guide.

STORY #87

Saints turn a deaf ear to praise. Praise makes us proud and careless. Bitter censure is the remedy for our faults, while sweet praise destroys our virtues. In the beginning, a devotee's aim is the realization of God. However, when people are attracted to him by his vows, rules, love of God, and his good conduct, he loses his purpose. This mass popularity leads him on the wrong path. Deceit, pride, and false shows of humility increase. By attaining the status of master, he loses forever his status as student. The result is the downfall of the saint.

THE HOLY MAN'S ADVICE

ONCE A HOLY MAN advised a devotee of truth: "Brother, be like a stone by the side of the road. As you are kicked about by pedestrians, your pride will disappear."

But then on second thought, the holy man felt that something was wrong with his advice. Yes, it's good that one should become like a stone, but what about the feet of the pedestrians? Wouldn't they be injured? So he modified his advice.

"Brother, be as humble as the dust on the street."

But then again he thought about his advice. He remembered that dust settles on the body and clothes of people and makes them dusty. So he finally said,

"Brother, be as cool as the moonbeam and bestow your calmness on others and make them happy."

Good men try to hide their virtues and bad men try to hide their vices, but neither virtue nor vice can be hidden long. How can one conceal the perfume of flowers in a beautiful garden, or the putrid smell of a rotten corpse in a ditch? We should admit our faults and be rid of them. An individual who cannot do without praise is like a cripple who cannot walk without crutches.

Story #88

Love has two characteristics: surrender and service. In the same way that whiteness, liquidity, and sweetness are the inseparable characteristics of milk, surrender and service are inseparable from love. This means that we should live for a beloved person or for others, not for ourselves. This is the supreme and infallible way to achieve happiness. When we enter the heart of our beloved and we allow our beloved into our heart, oneness occurs, and this oneness is called love. Surrender and service to each other then become so subtle they are almost invisible.

The Story of Divarka and Kalpalata

ONCE THERE WAS A young man named, Divarka. One day his two uncles called him to their sides and said, "Divarka, it's time for you to get married. We've found you a bride."

Divarka sat silently for a few minutes with downcast eyes. At last he spoke, in a low, unhappy voice.

"I know you both want only what's best for me. You've raised me since the death of my parents right up to this present moment. You've educated me properly. You've helped me attain a temporary job. But wouldn't it be more beneficial for me to wait two years until I'm more established with my job before marrying?"

"We agree with you," his uncles said. "It would be best to wait. But we like this bride very much and who knows, two years from now we may not be able to find a girl with such good character."

Divarka agreed and three days later he got married.

He liked his new wife very much. He was impressed by her thoughts, speech, and behavior.

"Uncles," he said a short time later. "You made a wise choice for me. Kalpalata is a pearl. She has transformed my whole life."

After five years, Divarka and Kalpalata had become one. Their minds were like two notes in perfect harmony. They had a three-year-old son and although they didn't live in luxury, their family was not in material want and they were rich with the wealth of love.

But then tragedy struck. Divarka worked for a food merchant and there was a fire in the shop and his employer lost millions of rupees. Two months later, his employer was killed in a car accident and Divarka lost his job altogether. He searched relentlessly for work, but was unable to find anything suitable.

If they had a little bit of grain to eat now, they couldn't afford a vegetable to go with it. They simply had no money for their basic needs. So Kalpalata secretly worked on the side. She was able to make a few rupees to keep the family from starving, but she never complained.

"Tell me the truth," Divarka said one day. "When was the last time you've eaten?"

Kalpalata laughed,

"Three days ago," she said, but it was a false laugh.

Tears rolled down Divarka's face and Kalpalata wiped them with her sari.

"Don't be sad," she said. "For a long time I've wanted to do a water fast and chant japa. Now I have the chance. You'll find work; I'm sure of it."

Divarka received consolation and hope from Kalpalata's words.

"Do you believe me?" She asked.

"If you want me to believe, then I believe," Divarka replied.

"No, I want to know if you believe!"

"Yes, I believe," Divarka said.

"Then listen to me," Kalpalata said. "I have gold jewelry worth 2000 rupees. Sell the jewelry and open a small shop."

Divarka was shocked.

"How could I ever sell your jewelry? I'll think about it and tell you tomorrow."

"No," Kalpalata said. "There's nothing to think about. Am I not yours? And if I'm yours, then my jewelry is yours, too. For the sake of our family, sell the jewelry. After you become successful, you can replace it."

Divarka agreed.

Within three months, his shop prospered. Soon he had to add on to the small building and he built two new rooms to handle the increased business. Within two years, he became a famous merchant. He approached the rich man who had bought Kalpalata's jewelry and the man still had the jewelry and Divarka bought it back, every piece of the original jewelry.

Four happy years went by. Then tragedy struck again. Kalpalata became mentally ill. She became worse and worse and finally totally deranged. She didn't speak anymore, but sat like a stone withdrawn into herself. She was neither conscious nor unconscious. She lost control of her bladder and bowels and she excreted all over the house.

Divarka bathed her and cleaned her soiled clothing and dressed her and sat with her every day. He lovingly fed her and put her to bed. His family and friends were deeply touched, but nonetheless they gave him unsolicited advice.

"Divarka," they said. "Place Kalpalata in an asylum. She can live peacefully there under the supervision of doctors and you can have you life back. You, too, will go mad if you keep living like this."

Moreover he was rich now and each person had someone for him to marry, someone in their own family, so they could share in his wealth.

Finally his closest friend approached him.

"Divarka," he said. "Enough is enough. Why are you making your life so miserable? Place your wife in an asylum and get married a second time."

"I can't do that," Divarka replied, deeply from his heart. "She's the reason why I'm successful. Furthermore she never abandoned me, not during my darkest moments, not during my unhappy days. She's still the same Kalpalata to me, sick or not. If I abandon her now when she needs me, there wouldn't be a more despicable man on earth."

His friend left, purified by Divarka's devotion, and no one gave him advice again.

Almighty God is love. Surrender and Service are His two Holy feet, and His feet purify us all. We humbly pray to Almighty God that He be compassionate and purify us all.

STORY #89

*A person can fulfill ordinary desires within a day, a month, or a
year. But to fulfill extraordinary desires, we must strive for innumerable lifetimes. A weak obstacle can destroy a weak thought, but
even the greatest obstacle can't destroy a bhavana, a strong thought
or conviction. When we use mantra to feed out thoughts, we create
an ocean of energy and strength.*

CHANTING RAM MADE THE BOULDERS FLOAT

ONCE RAVANA, THE KING of Lanka, kidnapped Lord Ram's
holy wife, Sita. When Lord Ram discovered this, he and
his army of monkeys set out to free her. They were soon
confronted with the vast barrier of the ocean which lay between
them and Lanka. Since there was no means of crossing the water, the most ingenious monkeys huddled for a discussion. After
thinking things over, they decided to build a bridge even though
they were fully aware that this would be a tremendous task for the
ocean was vast. However, when the most clever monkeys presented this problem to the full assembly, the others were undaunted by
this challenge. All the monkeys said,

"There's no problem here. We'll construct the bridge in a matter of days."

The leaders were pleased by the enthusiasm of everyone under
their command.

The army woke up the next day well before dawn. After
quickly finishing their morning routine, they went right to work
building the bridge. All the monkeys chanted the mantra, 'Ram,'
as they carried boulders toward the ocean. Their love was so strong
that huge boulders weighing many tons seemed to weigh only few
pounds. Totally absorbed in building the bridge, they didn't notice
whether it was night or day. As they continued to chant Ram's
name, the power of their love for the Lord carried the boulders
across the surface of the ocean, just as if they were dry leaves.

Lord Ram had been watching the construction from a distance. When he saw boulders floating with the support of nothing but the name, Ram, he was astonished. Rocks always sink but these were floating! He was forced to believe the evidence before his eyes. They were floating on the strength of the mantra, Ram. Yet he, himself, was Ram and he found it hard to believe that the monkeys were performing this task simply with the support of his name.

"Where did this divine strength in his name come from?" He asked.

He decided to test it himself. So early the next morning, Lord Ram went covertly to the seashore.

Just as a master always knows the temperament of his devoted servant, a servant always knows his master's temperament. The supremely valiant, Hanuman, had seen Lord Ram watching the bridge construction and had immediately guessed Ram's intentions. So Hanuman trailed him secretly to the seashore.

Lord Ram picked up a small stone from the shore and placed it on the ocean's surface. Immediately it sank. Yet tons of boulders placed by the monkeys had floated. His small stone sank.

"How can there be power in my name, but no power in me, the person bearing that name?" He asked puzzled.

Then Hanuman, the most clever of all the monkeys, came out from hiding behind a tree and bowed down to him. Lord Ram broke into laughter, despite his embarrassment, for he realized that clever Hanuman had seen his experiment.

"Lord Ram," Hanuman said with a smile, "When I saw you watching the bridge construction, I guessed that you would want to see if you, too, could make a stone float. So I followed you to the seashore today."

"My dear, Hanuman," Lord Ram asked innocently. "Why did my stone sink?"

"My Lord," Hanuman replied, "Anything in the ocean of the world that you abandon must sink. Although you're Lord Ram, himself, you don't know the importance of your own name because you're beyond feeling self-important. The monkeys, however, are your sincere devotees and to them your name is important. How can nectar know its own sweetness? The taste can be appreciated only by the taster. Superficially, it might seem that this miracle is due to the monkey's firm faith, but the miracle is due to your grace. Faith without the support of your grace is powerless."

The unique feature of saintliness is that whoever has this quality is completely unaware that he is a saint. Just as flowers silently exude their fragrance and a lamp silently gives light, flowers in the form of saints silently spread the fragrance of restraint and character. Miracles manifested through them are always genuine miracles. Through such miracles we become aware of the reality of divine energy. Just as electricity amazes everyone who sees it working through an inert object, the energy working through a saint is also amazing. Material scientists have accomplished clairvoyance by inventing the television and clairaudience by inventing the radio. Unaided by these devices, however, the spiritual scientists use powers generated from yogic disciplines. They can see distant objects by the power of clairvoyance and can hear distant sounds by the power of clairaudience. The material scientist directs his efforts toward the non-soul, away from his Atman The spiritual scientist directs his efforts towards his Atman One is a child-yogi. The other is a mature yogi.

STORY #90

You all chant the Vishnu mantra, Om Namo Bhagavate
Vasudevaya, to purify your mind and body. Be sure to repeat it
sincerely. If you practice this japa in the best possible way, you
will purify your body and mind, and the feeling of surrender will
flourish in you.

This mantra, and others such as Gayatri, Ram, and Om, are
mantras of divine origin. They have all evolved from anahat nad.
The simple letters, words, and sentences which form these mantras
aren't as simple as they seem. They have special energy hidden in
them and grant wonderful blessings to the seeker.

Dadaji, Why Chant Mantra Repeatedly?

ONCE MY REVEREND GURUDEV instructed me to chant the mantra, Om Namah Shivaya, so I did as he said. After about 1,000 repetitions, however, it occurred to me that although the mantra means, I bow to You, Lord Shiva, I wasn't bowing to Lord Shiva. My tongue was merely saying, Om Namah Shivaya, Om Namah Shivaya, Om Namah Shivaya...I bow to You, Lord Shiva. I bow to You, Lord Shiva. I bow to You, Lord Shiva. Yet, I wasn't able to comprehend the mantra's secret.

Then another thought came to me. Why repeat the sentence, I bow to You, over and over? Why can't I just tell the Lord this once and be done with it? Why should I repeat the same sentence millions and billions of times? Wouldn't the listener become tired of hearing it?

Becoming impatient with these thoughts, I put down my mala and ran and bowed at the holy feet of my Gurudev.

"Gurudev," I said. I'm chanting the mantra, Om Namah Shivaya, according to your instructions, but I haven't once bowed down to Lord Shiva! Should I bow to Him each time I speak the mantra, or should I bow to Him over and over without saying the mantra? This repeated bowing down should be called, bowing japa!"

In a serious, but affectionate voice, he replied,

"Son, your statement is correct from one point of view, but it's incorrect from another. Yes, it's true that the literal meaning of the words, Om Namah Shivaya, is, I bow to You, Lord Shiva, but the intended meaning is totally different. The intended meaning is, I surrender to You, Lord Shiva."

"But Gurudev," I asked, "Why should I keep reminding Lord Shiva that I've surrendered to Him? Couldn't I just tell Him once? Why should I repeat the same sentence so many times?"

"Here, too, you're mistaken," Gurudev explained. "The Lord is very compassionate. If we tell Him just once, I surrender to You, He accepts it immediately. But the chanter's mind is distracted and it escapes somewhere else right after speaking the mantra. His mind moves his mouth in rote repetition of the words, but doesn't sincerely surrender. In order for the distracted mind to become pure and sincerely surrender to the Lord, the seeker must repeat the mantra thousands and thousands of times. The labor of so many mantra repetitions succeeds when the mind finally sincerely accepts the idea of surrender and becomes so concentrated that it becomes no-mind. At that point, without mind, who needs japa?"

STORY #91

THE DULL SILVERSMITH

ONCE THERE WAS A rich man. He had one son. The rich man died and left his fortune to his son, but his son squandered the fortune and became poor. The only things the son had left were a silver image of Lord Shiva and a silver image of Nandi, a male cow.

One day he had to sell even these images of God. They were made of silver, so he visited a silversmith. The silversmith weighed the image of Lord Shiva and also the image of Nandi.

"I'll give you 300 rupees for the image of Lord Shiva and 500 rupees for the image of Nandi." he said.

The son was still a devotee of God. He had been raised in a spiritual home, even though he had squandered his wealth. To him the image of Lord Shiva was far more valuable than the image of Nandi, because he saw these objects in terms of their spiritual value.

"Kind sir," he said. "You have it wrong. The image of Lord Shiva should be worth 500 rupees and the image of Nandi, his vehicle, should be worth 300 rupees."

"No!" the silversmith replied. "I don't see these objects as Shiva and Nandi. I see only the silver in them."

We are all like that sometimes. We see only the silver in this world and not God.

STORY #92

THE FORGETFUL HUSBAND

ONCE THERE WAS A loving husband who was very forgetful. He forgot everything. It didn't matter what it was,
he just forgot it.

One day he died. A few weeks later the doctor who had cared
for him visited his widow and family. The doctor was kind and
wanted to see if the family was alright. But then he got serious.

"Sister," he said. "Why did your husband die? I've wondered
about this for two weeks. I cared for him during his last days, but
I can't figure out why he died. He had a few minor illnesses, but
nothing serious."

"I know why he died," the woman replied. "My husband was
very forgetful. He forgot to breath. I'm sure of it. That's why he
died."

STORY #93

THE FORGETFUL PROFESSOR

O NCE THERE WAS A brilliant professor who was also very forgetful. One day he was walking home from the university where he taught and it started to rain. He opened his umbrella and continued walking home.

He decided that as soon as he got home he was going to hang his umbrella on a peg near the door and lie down and take a nap. When he arrived home, his wife was gone. He was so forgetful that he placed his umbrella on the bed and went and stood under the peg near the door.

We are all like that sometimes. We are very forgetful. We remember only those things that please us. God is not as pleasing to us as the things of the world, and so we forget God.

STORY #94

I Am Still the Same Person

AFTER MY SANYAS INITIATION, I started traveling along the shores of the Narmada River. Usually, I never spent more than a day or two in any one village. Moreover, I used to stay in a temple or in an inn outside the village. Shri Gurudev Shantanandji Maharji, who gave me sanyas initiation, had given me two dhotis, two kurtas, several loincloths, a towel, a bed sheet, a blanket, a mat, and other necessary items. Since I was a novice sanyasi, I was burning with the spirit of renunciation. For two or three months afterwards, I carried my belongings on my shoulders.

One day, I was walking along the shores of the Narmada. It occurred to me that the clothes that I was wearing were adequate. Extra clothes seemed superfluous. Since I had renounced the world, I felt it was improper to cling to extra possessions. I reflected on this for a while, and then I simply loosened the grip on the bundle I was carrying on my back. I didn't even bother to look behind me to see where it fell. But this action was prompted by my lack of prior experience.

Later, I began some constructive tasks in the village. Often, due to their strong insistence, I had to stay in the homes of the householders. I soon realized that whenever I had to wash my one and only kurta, I would have only a loincloth to wear around the house. So, I was obliged to add another kurta plus two or three other garments to my belongings.

People used to invite me to their meals, and I would arrive daily at the appointed lunchtime. At such times, I used to sit on an ordinary mat or on whatever was put down for me. When nothing was laid, I used to sit on the bare ground. To me, the love of my hosts was of primary importance. The mat and other luxuries were secondary.

As my name and fame spread, society began to respect me more and more. Ordinary mats gradually disappeared and were replaced by more comfortable mats, backrests, and silken bed sheets. Usually, I traveled on foot, but whenever someone arranged for a vehicle, I would ride.

There was a gradual change in this situation also. Villagers began to provide me with private vehicles and a private residence. Some of those luxuries I liked, and some I didn't. However, since I was cooperating with other people's wishes, these situations were pleasant for them.

And yet, my mind was constantly stuck with one pain: that I was gradually becoming distant from these simple people who had provided me with ordinary mats. They were beginning to believe that I was becoming a lover of luxuries. But a sanyasi has to move within different classes of society and he is expected to live in accordance with the way each class lives. Yet, an old group of devotees always dislikes new arrangements, and new groups always dislike the old arrangements. I have continually tried to find a solution to this problem; yet, I have not succeeded.

Moreover, in the formative years of my sanyasi life, my secluded activities of sadhana, writing, and reading were done to a minimum extent. Thus, I was able to give more of my time to society. But now, if any person wants to see me, he has to make an appointment well ahead of time. In spite of this, he hardly gets five or ten minutes with me. Many people dislike this arrangement. With all my heart, I can only say that I am the same person now that I was years ago. There has not been any change in my love or personality. And yet, due to changing times and circumstances, I appear to be an offender to people.

STORY #95

Don't look upon the faults of others. By doing so, your own consciousness will become impure. If you hold something dirty and stinking in your hand, what happens? Your hand will stink, too. When you dwell on the faults of others, you dirty your mind. If you must dwell on faults, dwell on your own faults. And if someone points out your faults, try to bear it and change.

SAINT TUKARAM AND HIS WIFE

ONCE IN INDIA THERE was a high saint named Tukaram. His wife loved to quarrel.

Whenever he chanted, "Ram, Ram," or, "Krishna, Krishna," she got irritated and stood in front of him and mocked him.

"Ram! Ram! Krishna! Krishna! What's all this nonsense? You're a worldly man, not a saint! Why do you chant these names all the time, as if you were a saint?"

But Tukaram would simply continue chanting.

Finally one day his wife got sick of it and left the house for awhile.

Later that same day, a devotee who considered Tukaram a saint, invited him to visit his sugarcane field. Tukaram politely refused, but the devotee insisted, so Tukaram visited the field.

When it was time for Tukaram to return home, the devotee cut fifteen sugarcanes, bound them into a bundle, and gave them to Tukaram. When the children of the village saw Tukaram walking by with a sugarcane bundle, they all wanted a piece. It was like candy to them.

"Tukadada!" They called, which means Grandfather Sugarcane. "Give us sugarcane!"

So Tukaram cut pieces for all the children he met.

When he arrived home, he had only one piece of sugarcane left. His wife immediately started a fight.

"You walked all the way into the country and you only brought back one piece of sugarcane? What's the matter with you?"

"Take it," Tukaram said, handing it to her. "You can have it."

She took it and banged him over the head with it and the sugarcane broke into two pieces.

"One for you and one for me," Tukaram said calmly.

What patience! He never saw his wife's faults. And he wasn't a weak husband.

"I chose to get married," he reasoned. "How can there be fault with my wife?"

This is the thought line of a devotee.

STORY #96

Our path is each our own; it is unique to us. We shouldn't try to imitate anyone. We shouldn't be like sheep that follow each other blindly. One by one sheep follow each other with their heads down, just looking at the tail and legs of the one in front of them, certain the one in the front is making all the right decisions. Yes, eventually we may choose a spiritual teacher and try to imitate that person, but we should study their character first for a long time, and select a teacher only if we think the person is right for us, not because they have a large following. Stay alert, guard your consciousness, and don't imitate anything unless you're convinced it's good for you.

THE POOR MAN AND HIS FANCY SUIT

ONCE THERE WAS A rich man. Over time, however, he became poorer and poorer. But he was an honest gentleman, so even though he was poor now, he was still invited to all the gatherings of the rich people in town.

He had saved one special suit for this purpose. It was exceptionally beautiful and stylish, and this was all he had left from his wealthy days. He knew he couldn't attend such functions dressed in poor clothes, so this is why he had saved the suit.

One evening he was getting ready to attend one of these gatherings and his wife said,

"The moths have eaten a hole in the sleeve of your suit! You can't go like this."

So she took out a needle and thread and made a very artistic patch over the hole. The patch was beautiful, truly striking.

That evening all the rich people were attracted to the suit.

"Where did you get that beautiful design?" They asked.

"My wife made it," the man said. "She designs clothes."

The next time they had a meeting everybody's suit had the same patch on it! At first there was a reason for the patch, then people just copied it. This happens in religion, too.

STORY #97

TOO MANY CLOTHES

IN THE EARLY DAYS when I traveled in the state of non-attachment, I used to bathe in rivers and lakes. I would wash my clothes by pounding them on nearby rocks. Since I didn't accept money from anyone, I was unable to buy soap. Usually, however, one of the local sisters would take the clothes that I had hung on a line, wash them again in the river with soap, and return them to the line.

After beginning my yoga sadhana, I used to stay in the homes of my disciples. They began to press my clothes daily. Feeling embarrassed, I would ask them not to do this, but expressing their helplessness they would tell me,

"Bapuji, the children are fighting among themselves to press your clothes and will not listen to us."

I would then motion them to sit close to me, and I would say,

"My children, we sanyasis are required to observe certain restrictions. What you may consider a service, someone else may think is a luxury."

They would then present their logic to me.

"Whoever comes here is coming only for your darshan. No one comes here to see whether you are wearing pressed or unpressed clothes. Stop being so concerned about what others think. You never asked us to press your clothes. If you had made such a request, we would never have pressed them."

I have learned to become tolerant in such matters.

After the ashrams of Malav and Kayavarohan were formed, my non-attachment became displeased with me and left me. Heaps and heaps of dhotis, kurtas, sweaters, shawls, towels, napkins, handkerchiefs, sandals, and shoes began to pile up. Whenever a brother or sister disciple would bring newly made clothes, I would lovingly scold them.

"Why have you gone through the trouble of sewing all these clothes without asking me first?"

"We don't need your instructions in such mundane matters," they would say.

"But I have many clothes," I would say.

"That's okay. We'll simply give them to some needy person. You don't have to be concerned about the matter."

I have never had time to reflect upon my worthiness or unworthiness. Whatever time I have had, I have used it to analyze and relish the loving feelings of my disciples. It is my strong desire also to remain steadfast on this path of love. Love is the most pious pilgrimage. Purity is acquired only by bathing in it.

STORY #98

THE MIRROR

IN 1948, I WAS giving discourses on the Gita in Halol, Amrit
Desai's birthplace. The assembly hall in which I was speaking was large. There was a small side room in which I lived.
This building was regularly used for gymnastics, and the equipment was usually stored in my room. When this equipment was
removed for my stay, however, a large mirror was inadvertently
left behind.

When I arrived there on the appointed day, the room was ready
for me. I could readily see that all the appropriate arrangements
had been made for my comfort. Then, my eyes fell on the huge
mirror. At that time, I practiced exercises regularly, but I had no
need of a mirror during practices.

It occurred to me that the mirror would have been protected
better if it had been stored elsewhere. Yet, I didn't question anyone about its presence in the room, for I assumed that the organizers had no need to use it elsewhere.

At that time I had not begun my yoga sadhana. My daily routine included praying, chanting mantra and hymns, and practicing
ordinary meditation. For this purpose I used to ask for two small
wooden platforms. I used one as a bench and the other as a table
for my ghee lamp. To keep the mirror safe from breaking, I placed
it on the platform with the lamp.

After my stay in Halol, I was supposed to go to Malav. It was
to have been my first visit there. Today, there is Kripalu Ashram
in Malav, but it wasn't established until much later. A gentleman
came from Malav to consult with the organizers in Halol about
making proper arrangements for my impending visit.

He was told,

"Take a pen and paper to his room and make a list of all the
things which are there. Arrange everything in Malav the way it is

arranged here. If you have any other questions, please come back and I'll try to help you.

Satisfied, he made a list of all the things which were required. When I went to Malav, I also found a mirror on one of the wooden platforms in my room. I was going to ask to have it taken away, but then I decided that it wasn't important enough to make a fuss about.

I appeared to be haunted by a large mirror wherever I went. When I arrived at the next village on my itinerary, Eral, there was a mirror waiting for me on its accustomed platform in my room. From that day on, I decided to give instructions each time I went to a new village not to have a mirror put in my room.

In Eral, I was a guest at the home of Thakor Saheb. He had arranged to place a very beautiful ivory-framed mirror in my room. Surely, he must have wondered how I was using this mirror. At first, he must have thought that I spent time sitting in front of this mirror contemplating my own form. Then, he must have dismissed the thought as being inappropriate. Eventually, he decided to ask me directly. One day, when we were both sitting in private, he remembered to ask the question.

"Gurudev," he said. "I have tried to arrive at a reasonable answer to this question, but I have not been satisfied. So, I'm asking you directly. If my question appears disrespectful to you, please don't answer it. Why do you keep a huge mirror on the wooden platform in your room?"

I broke into laughter and said,

"Brother, this mirror business has been haunting me ever since I once made a mistake!"

Then I narrated the entire sequence of events to him.

STORY #99

Yama and niyama build a person's character so thoroughly that by sincerely practicing them one ceases to be an animal, grows into a real human being, and can even transform into the Lord. Although their practice is arduous, fear of failure is unwarranted, because we are only required to practice yama and niyama to the best of our capacity.

THE LABORER AND THE THREE STONES

A RICH MAN WAS building a temple on the summit of a high mountain. He needed to have three large stones carried up the mountainside. After deciding how much he would pay for the labor, the rich man gave the task to a certain laborer.

The laborer was strong, and he eagerly started up the mountain carrying all three stones at once. After climbing for awhile, however, he became tired and felt the need to lighten his load. He left one stone on a ledge and continued climbing with the two remaining stones.

However after climbing for a distance, he felt the need to lighten his load even more. So, he left the second stone on another ledge. After that his load was much lighter, and within his carrying capacity. He was able to successfully complete his task.

Be patient. Love the Lord. Life is very, very difficult. We will inevitably make mistakes. Pray to the divine beings for mercy: "Lord, You are my entire life. You be my guard. Stay in my heart. Stay in my eyes. I have no other answer, than this prayer: Merciful One, keep your merciful eyes upon me."

STORY #100

FANNING THE GURU

YEARS AGO WHEN I was in India, a group of disciples in a village once invited me to give a lecture. So, I went there for a few days. At the home of my host, I was seated on a high platform. In front of me sat disciples and other devoted villagers. Two sentimental disciples were standing on either side of me fanning me.

The tradition of fanning one's guru is a well-established one in every village in India. As a result, those who organize the lectures usually arrange to have fans available. If for some reason, this arrangement is neglected, some experienced person is sure to feel the absence. He then arranges to have fans brought.

The saint is supposed to be kept cool whether the temperature is high or not. As a result, the saint grows in love and tolerance. Devotees who are fanning are not merely fanning; they are expressing all the love in their heart. During such situations, many times I have said to my devotees, young and old,

"Your arms will get tired."

Usually they reply affectionately,

"Our arms aren't tired. When they become tired, we'll put the fan aside."

At other times, I have said,

"I don't feel hot. It will be alright if you don't fan me."

At this they have answer,

"We're not fanning you. We're keeping the flies away."

I've responded hundreds of times,

"It's alright. There's no need to fan them away."

To this they reply,

"Well, you may not have a need, but we do. When we're fanning you, we're comforting ourselves with the thought that we're serving our Guruji. It's also a good excuse for us to stand beside you."

Those children then keep fanning me even when the electric ceiling fans are working.

I tell them,

"Two or three electric fans are already working. Why don't you rest?"

Then they frown and say,

"If we don't fan you, the elders will not allow us to sit near you. They'll shoo us away."

This fanning argument usually goes on at great length, but I've narrated it here briefly for you.

One day, upon seeing two brothers were fanning me very conscientiously, a devotee whispered into one of the disciple's ears,

"Is your Guru hot because he has drunk some potion or brew? Why do you fan him so vigorously?"

The criticized disciple wasn't able to tolerate these words. Immediately he came to me and complained about the incident.

I asked him to send the offending brother to me.

The brother came, bowed down, and then stood beside me. There was no negativity in his mind. After greeting him, I lovingly explained to him,

"Brother, I haven't had anything to drink. I don't feel hot, and I haven't instructed these two brothers to fan me constantly."

Then I suggested that the two brothers put the fans aside and sit down. They submitted to my request.

Darshan was the only activity planned. Groups of devotees would approach me, bow down, and then make way for another group of devotees. After a while, two people came, bowed down, then immediately reached for the fans and began to fan me.

Lovingly, I said,

"My dear brothers. I really don't feel hot, so why don't you please be seated?"

Again the fans were put aside.

Another group of devotees came forward. Two brothers from that group picked up the fans and began fanning.

The brother who had earlier criticized my being fanned soon realized that he had made a mistake in criticizing the matter. He came over and asked my forgiveness.

Hoping to comfort him, I patted his head and said,

"Since you have not committed any offense, it isn't necessary for me to pardon you. Fanning the guru is one of the well-established religious traditions in our country. Through it we can easily express our love and service. In large assemblies you would be amazed to see how many brothers and sisters rise to their feet one after another to fan me.

He smiled lovingly, bowed down, and returned to his seat.

Story #101

On the spiritual path, it's improper to ask questions as soon as they appear in our minds. This represents restlessness of the mind. Some questions only produce other questions, not answers. The mystery behind this, of course, is that there are different levels of questions.

On Grandfather's Lap

ONCE A SMALL CHILD was seated on his grandfather's lap. The child saw the white mustache on his grandfather.

"Grandfather," the child asked, playing with the mustache, "What's this?"

"It's called a mustache," the grandfather replied.

The child looked at the mustache for a while. He played with it a little longer. Then he thought of another question.

"Who has a mustache?" He asked.

"Fathers. Uncles. Older brothers," the grandfather replied. The child played with the mustache some more, twirling it around in his fingers. Then he thought of another question.

"Can my mother have a mustache?" He asked.

"No," the grandfather said. "Mothers don't have mustaches."

The child played with the mustache some more. Then he thought of another question.

"Why not?" He asked.

The grandfather thought for a moment. Then decided not to explain why mothers don't have mustaches. How would a small child understand it?

On the spiritual path, childish questions are not only asked by children, they are also asked by learned older people. The old and the learned ask childish questions if they are ignorant of the subject.

STORY #102

How to Chant OM

BEFORE YOU CHANT OM, you must relax and withdraw the energy, the outgoing energy, and focus it within. Then take a long, deep breath and chant the sound of OM.

Continue to say OM as long as you can with one breath. Then experience the vibrations that are generated within your body and mind.

Start another OM and let your mind dissolve in the sound. Then sit still and experience the vibrations generated within your body and mind again.

If you continue doing this with a peaceful, steady mind, you will experience peace, joy, and bliss.

OM is the king mantra; all the other mantras are included in it.

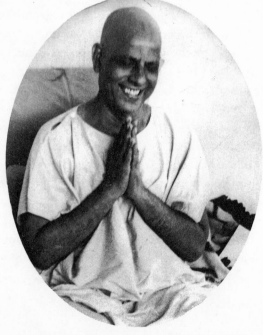